LIBRARY & INFORMATION SERVICE
ODSTOCK HOSPITAL
SALISBURY SP2 8BJ

To be renewed or returned on or before the date marked below:

07. APR 98		

PLEASE ENTER ON LOAN SLIP:

AUTHOR: MEALS, R.A.

TITLE: AN ATLAS OF FOREARM AND HAND
              CROSS-SECTIONAL ANATOMY

ACCESSION NO:	CLASS MARK:
1207	WE 640 460

An Atlas of
Forearm and Hand
Cross-Sectional Anatomy

An Atlas of
Forearm and Hand
Cross-Sectional Anatomy

with Computed Tomography and
Magnetic Resonance Imaging correlation

Roy A Meals
Associate Professor of Orthopaedic Surgery

Leanne L Seeger
Assistant Professor of Radiological Sciences

University of California, Los Angeles

MARTIN DUNITZ

© Roy A Meals and Leanne L Seeger 1991

First published in the United Kingdom in 1991
by Martin Dunitz Ltd., 7-9 Pratt Street, London NW1 0AE

A CIP catalogue record for this book is available from the
British Library.

ISBN 1-85317-029-1

Designed, illustrated and computer generated by
Marks Illustration and Design Consultants
Colour origination by Imago Publishing Ltd
Manufactured by Imago Publishing Ltd
Printed and bound in Singapore

To Susan, Clifton and Rudi
who help keep us on course

Contents

Foreword

Drs Meals and Seeger deserve our congratulations for their achievement in making this outstanding atlas of the forearm and hand. The work has been accomplished with admirable technical skill, based on originality and carried out with devotion.

I should like to emphasize again the importance of cross-sectional analysis, as I have always advocated in my teaching. It is the only way to study the spatial relations in the body without distortion. It can hardly be emphasized enough that anatomy is the science of spatial coherence within differentiated substrate related to functional activities, including development. Systemic units can be distinguished in the body, but the body cannot be considered to be composed of those units. This fundamental quality of anatomy or human morphology is shown best in cross-sectional anatomy and the non-invasive radiological modalities of CT and MRI.

It is most fortunate that owing to modern clinical methods a revival in cross-sectional anatomy can be observed. This can only enhance profitable exchange between the clinical sciences and fundamental morphology.

I would like to see this unique atlas in the hands of all those involved in the human hand – anatomists, radiologists and surgeons.

Johan M. F. Landsmeer
Emeritus Professor, Faculty of Medicine,
University of Leiden, The Netherlands

Introduction

Accurate maps facilitate careful explorations. Careful explorations facilitate accurate mapmaking. These interlocking tenets apply to ancient mariners, modern astronomers, and anatomists of all times. Sailors and astronomers explore and map without distorting their subjects, but unfortunately the same is not true for anatomists. In the course of studying precise relationships among structures, the anatomical relationships are disturbed. When diagnosis and treatment of anatomical derangements are crude, then precise delineations of the relationships are superfluous. Hand surgery, however, is continually becoming more sophisticated as are the indirect, non-invasive imaging techniques of computed tomography (CT) and magnetic resonance (MR) imaging. These imaging techniques allow for both good maps and careful exploration and demand the conceptualization of the anatomy in cross section. Furthermore, as treatments become less invasive and more specific with developments in arthroscopy, microsurgery, laser surgery, cryoprobes and so forth, the conventional layer-by-layer, superficial-to-deep anatomical maps provide insufficient detail for the modern explorer.

In the region of the forearm and hand, gross anatomy perhaps reaches its highest refinement since multiple distinct tissues of unique qualities are compactly arranged to form a versatile tool. That tool is a marvel of mechanical virtuosity, delicate sensibility and emotional sensitivity, yet its components are all grossly visible, and an understanding of their interworkings clearly explains the hand's versatility. This atlas aims to meet that growing need for detailed, undistorted yet direct mapping of anatomy in this complex and fascinating region.

The right upper limb used to prepare the cross-sectional photographs was obtained from a fifty-nine-year-old man of moderate build. Shortly after death, the axillary vessels were ligated and the limb removed through the proximal humerus. The limb was washed and shaved and then positioned in sand. The elbow was fully extended, the forearm fully supinated, the wrist placed in a neutral position, the thumb widely abducted and the fingers fully extended. The sand maintained the position during freezing and prevented pressure artifacts by widely distributing the weight. Once thoroughly frozen, the limb was removed from the sand. Several small areas of artifactual skin folds were locally thawed, smoothed and rapidly refrozen. Photographs and radiographs of the limb were obtained (pages 14-19). The limb was then carefully positioned in a rectangular wooden box using small heaps of crushed ice to keep the limb from contacting the box at any point. Once this construct was frozen solid and the accurate position of the limb verified, the box was filled completely with crushed ice. This minimized the remaining space to be filled with ice water and thereby the distortion as the water expanded from liquid to solid form during the final freeze.

A butcher-type band saw used for surgical pathology was especially adapted to make parallel, evenly spaced cuts across the end of the previously prepared ice block. Rubber scrapers were positioned on both sides of the saw blade at two levels to prevent the blade from depositing melted ice and tissue debris back on the cut surface of the ice block. The ice block was placed into a closely fitting, double walled trough which was securely clamped to the sliding portion of the band saw table. Dry ice was placed in the space between the walls to keep the ice block frozen during the sectioning. Turning a screw drive mechanism advanced the end of the ice block 3 mm before each pass through the saw, thereby providing a limb and ice section approximately 2 mm thick, with kerf loss accounting for the remaining thickness. The face of the ice block and frozen limb cross section was photographed before each pass through the saw by a camera clamped to the back edge of the band saw table. Thus the precise x-y orientation of each section with respect to the entire limb was preserved. The 2-mm-thick sections were placed horizontally on black vinyl cards and allowed to thaw at room temperature. The moisture from the melted ice was carefully blotted away and each thawed section was photographed on a copy stand. Two banks of tungsten 3400 lamps illuminated the specimens from 45-degree angles through polarizing filters. A polarizing filter on the camera lens was rotated until minimal glare was noted reflecting from the moist surface of the section. A Nikon camera set for automatic shutter speed at f11 through a 55 mm macro lens recorded the image on Kodak Ectakrome EPY 135 slide film. Thanks goes to Mike Kabo for his superhuman assistance on one very long, tedious Saturday of sectioning and photographing.

A 20 by 30-inch color poster print was made from the slide of each thawed section in order to study, identify and label structures as small as cutaneous nerves. The color prints in the atlas are taken from the original slides and are reproduced at life size. They are oriented appropriately in their x-y frames by matching their rotation to the corresponding photograph taken before the section was cut away from the ice block. By convention, the limb is viewed from distal to proximal, as if the viewer is standing at the body's foot looking toward the axilla.

For both the CT and MR images, the arm of a normal volunteer was positioned in a fashion identical to that used for freezing and sectioning the cadaver arm. CT images were acquired using a General Electric (GE) 9800 scanner. Contiguous 3 mm thick slices were obtained, using 2-second scans at 120 kV and 40 mA. Intravenous contrast was not infused. Medium-scan and 14-cm display fields-of-view were used. In order to maximize visualization of both bony and soft tissue structures, a window width of 500 and level of 80 were used for photography. MR images were acquired with a 1.5 Tesla GE Signa MR imaging system. Spin-echo T1-weighted techniques were used, with a repetition time (TR) of 600 msec, and a time-to-echo (TE) of 25 msec. Two signal averages were used, with an imaging matrix of 256 x 128. Imaging field-of-view was 14 cm. We would also like to thank the Tarzana Regional Hospital MRI Center for the use of their MR imaging system.

The page design places the CT image bottom left, below the color photograph, with the MR image bottom right. Because of the necessity of using different limbs for the various studies and because of slight differences in limb length, orientation and level of cut, precise correspondence of the structures at some levels are lacking. For the same reasons, some of the anatomical sections do not have accompanying CT or MR images. By studying the sections immediately proximal and distal to the level of interest, the missing information can be inferred.

Especial thanks go to the donor of the body used in this atlas. We hope that he would appreciate the irony that in the process of cutting his limb into several hundred pieces, its detailed, undistorted anatomy has been carefully preserved as an accurate map.

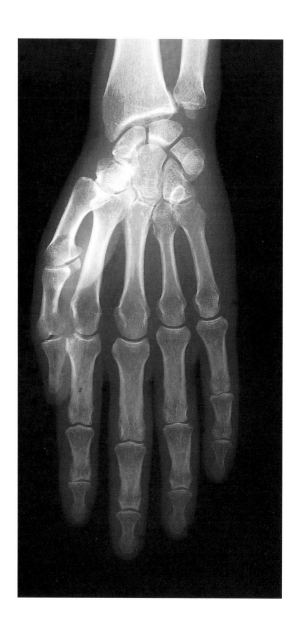

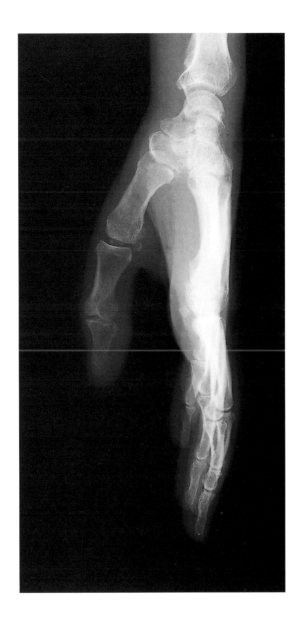

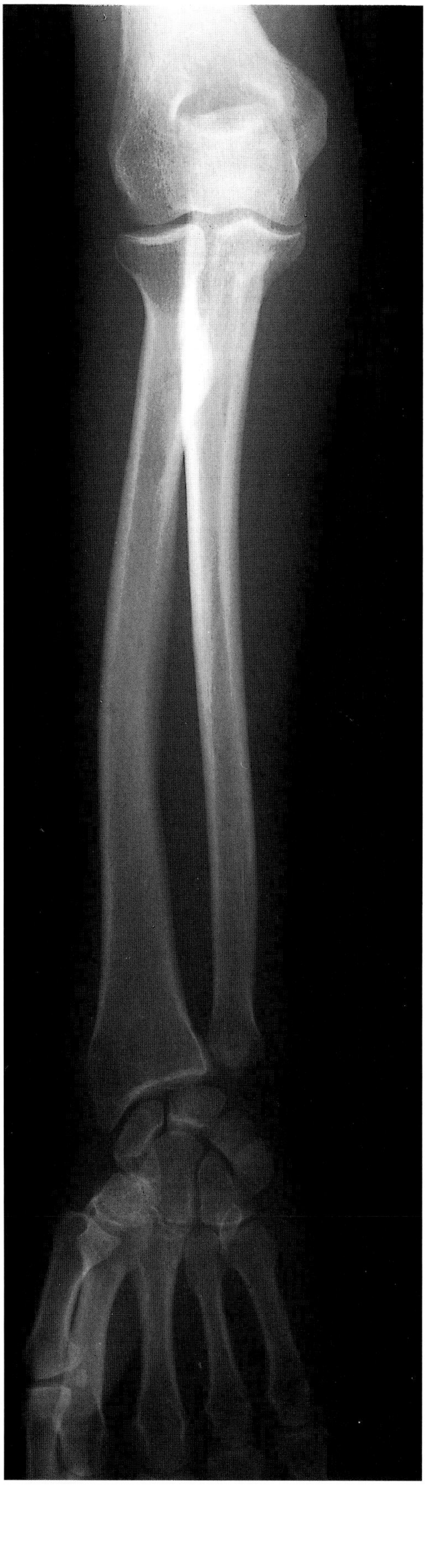

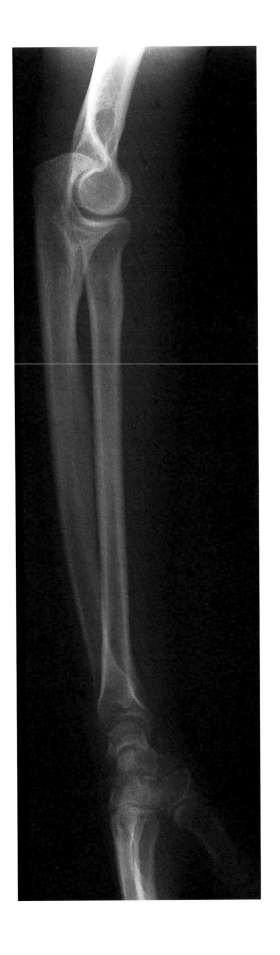

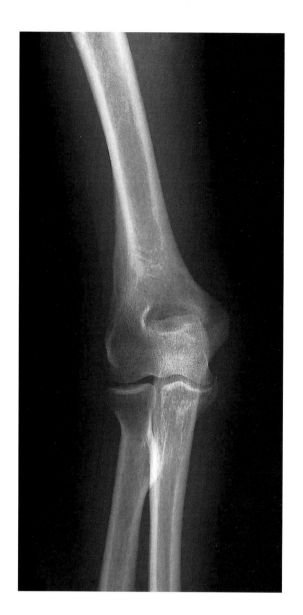

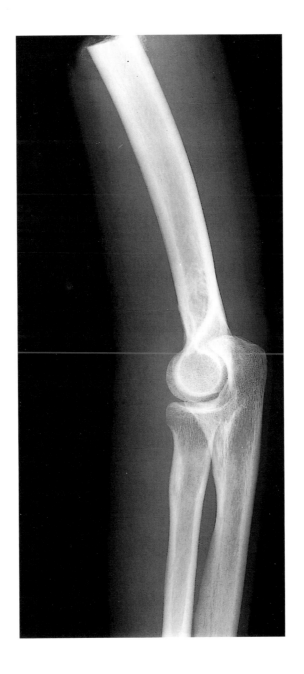

figure 1

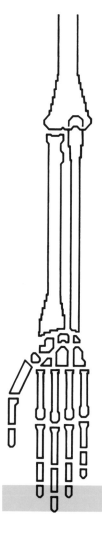

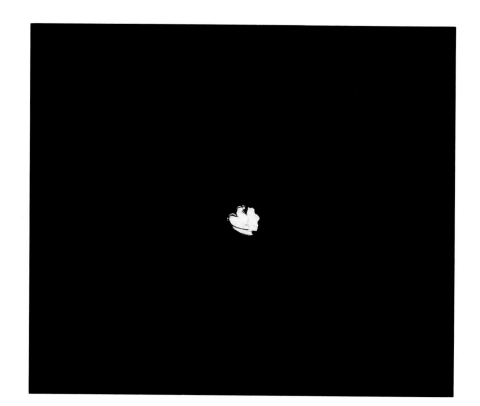

Tip middle finger

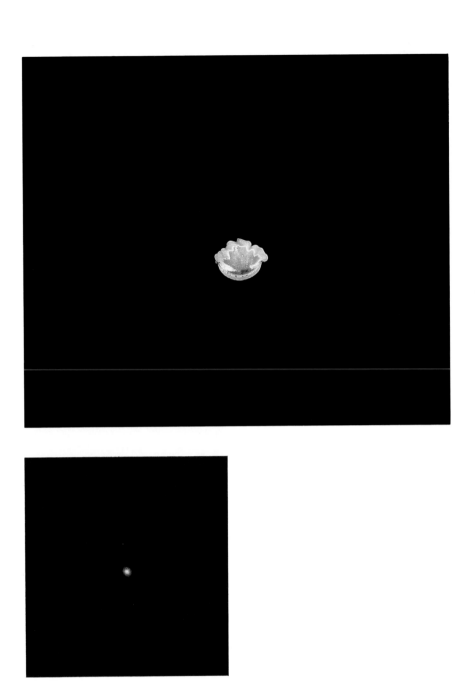

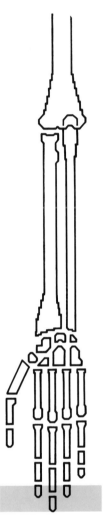

figure 2

figure 3

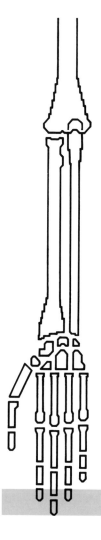

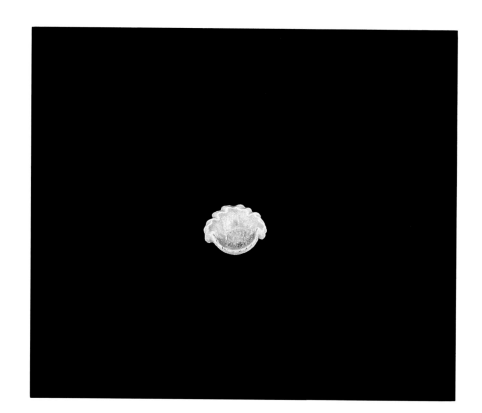

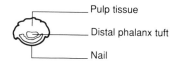

Pulp tissue

Distal phalanx tuft

Nail

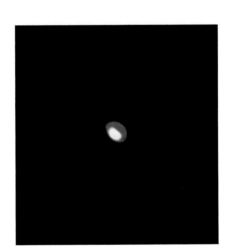

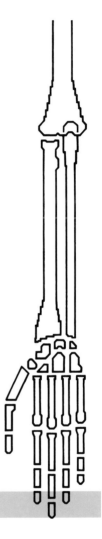

figure 4

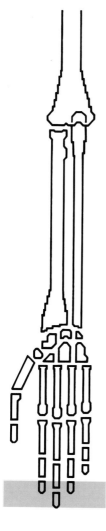

figure 5

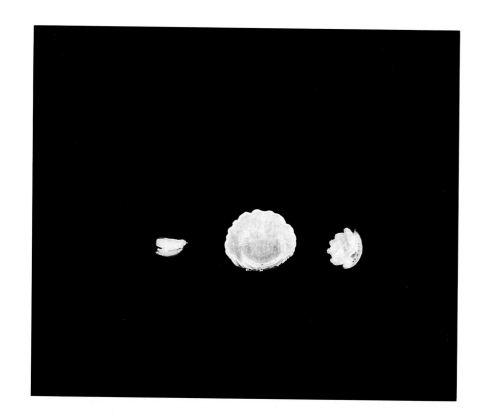

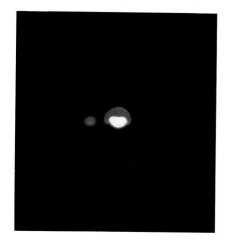

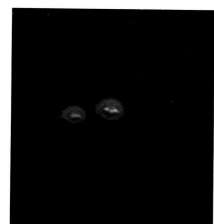

Tip index 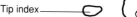 Tip ring finger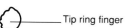

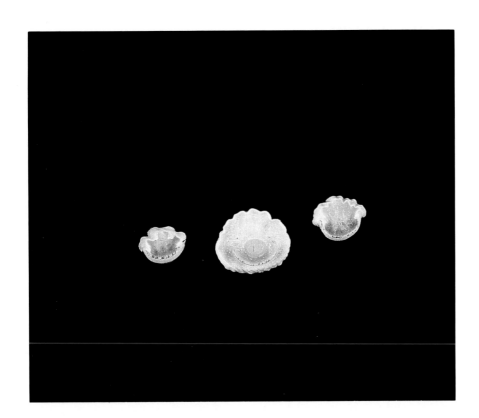

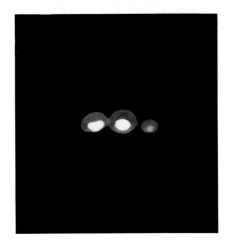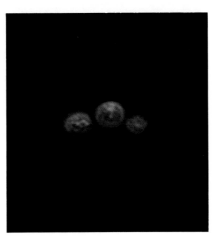

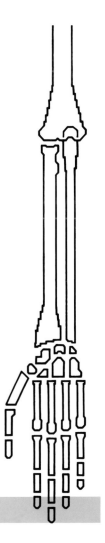

figure 6

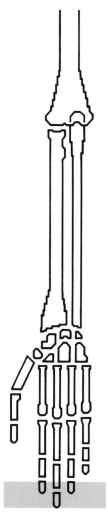

figure 7

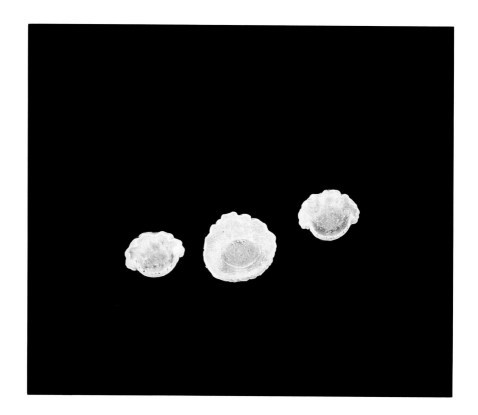

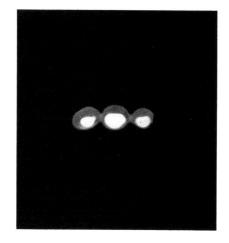

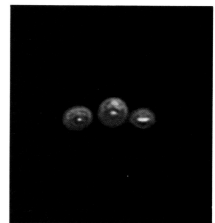

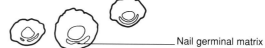

Nail germinal matrix

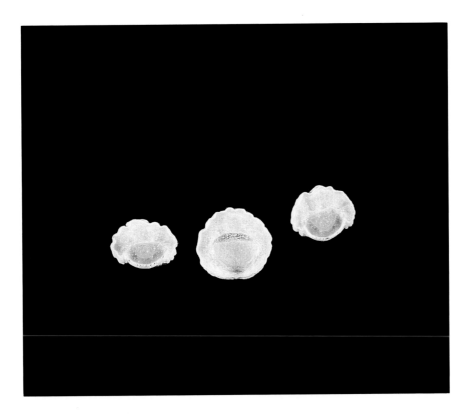

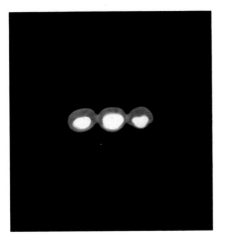

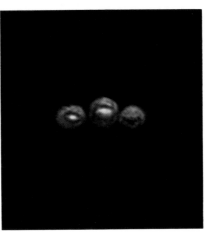

figure 8

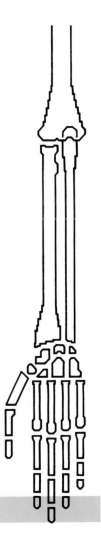

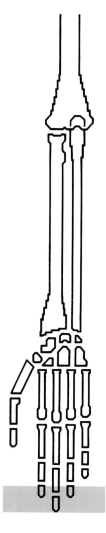

figure 9

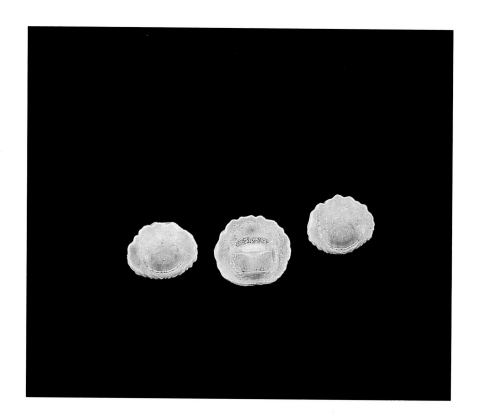

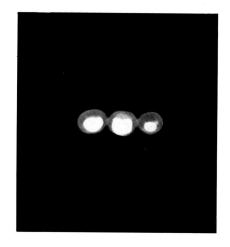

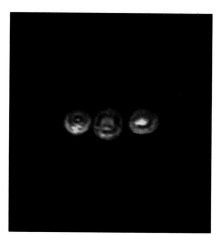

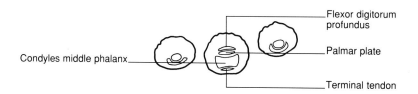

Condyles middle phalanx ———

——— Flexor digitorum profundus

——— Palmar plate

——— Terminal tendon

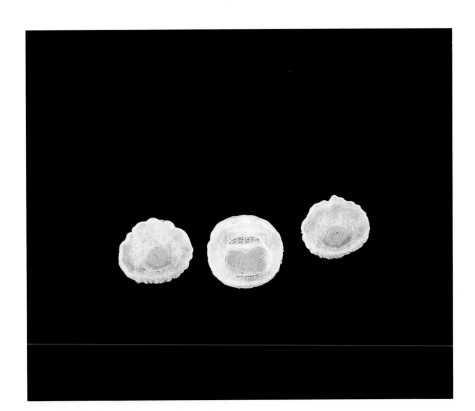

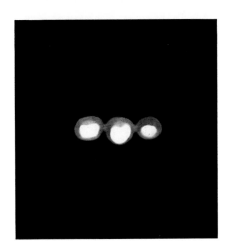

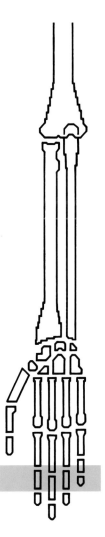

figure 10

figure 11

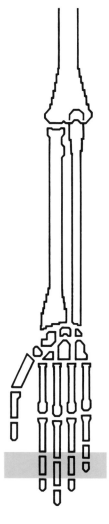

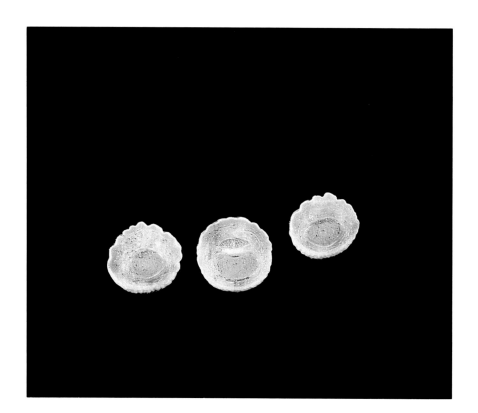

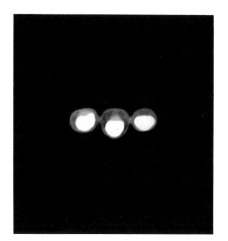

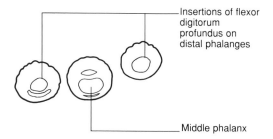

Insertions of flexor digitorum profundus on distal phalanges

Middle phalanx

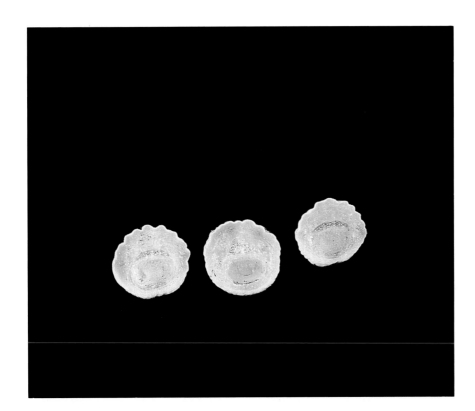

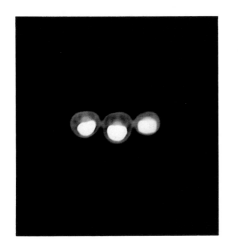

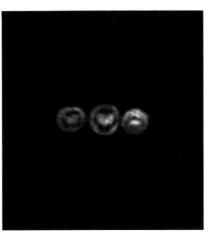

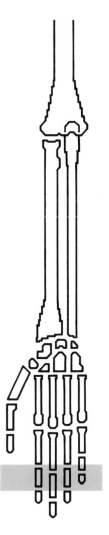

figure 12

figure 13

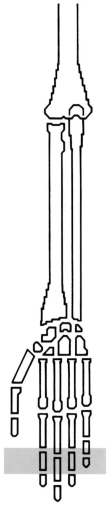

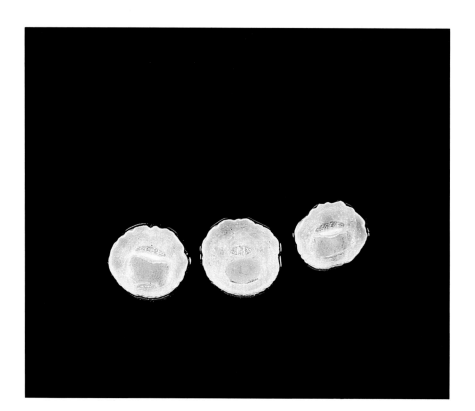

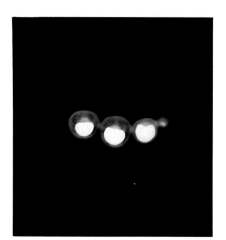

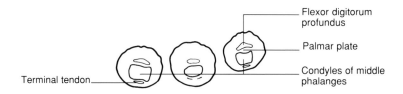

Flexor digitorum profundus

Palmar plate

Condyles of middle phalanges

Terminal tendon

figure 14

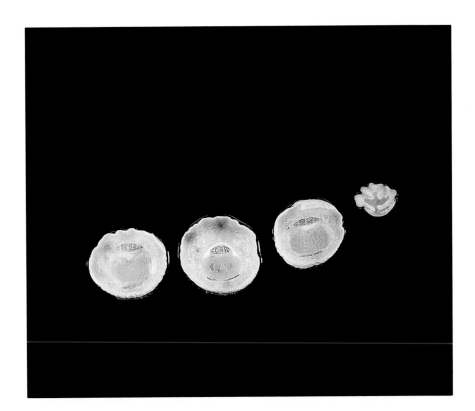

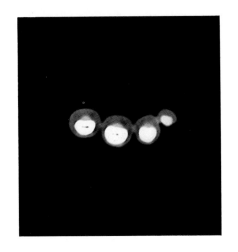

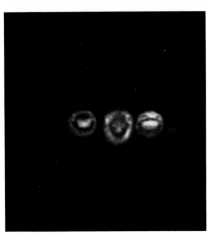

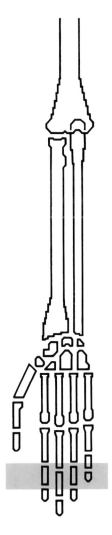

figure 15

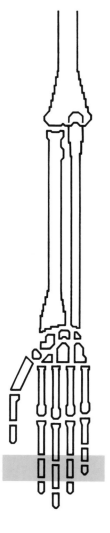

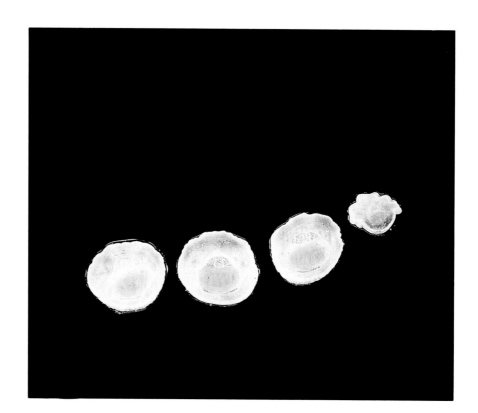

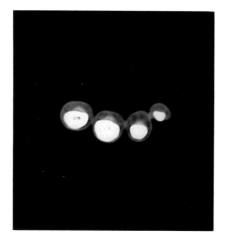
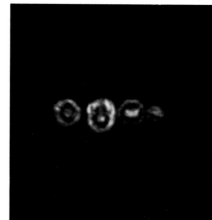

Flexor digitorum
superficialis insertion ——————————————

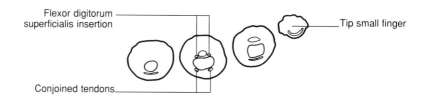

——— Tip small finger

Conjoined tendons ————

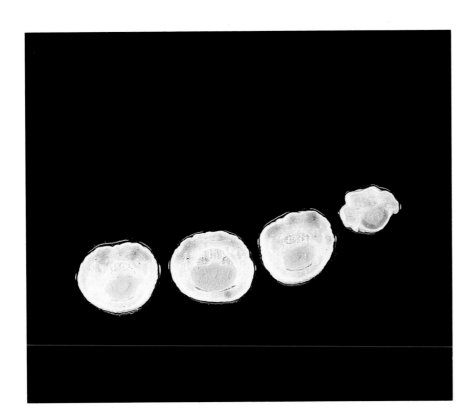

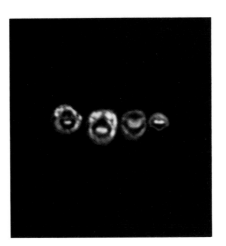

figure 16

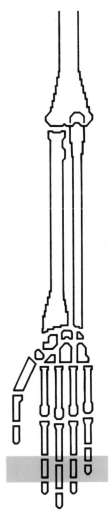

figure 17

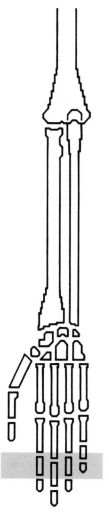

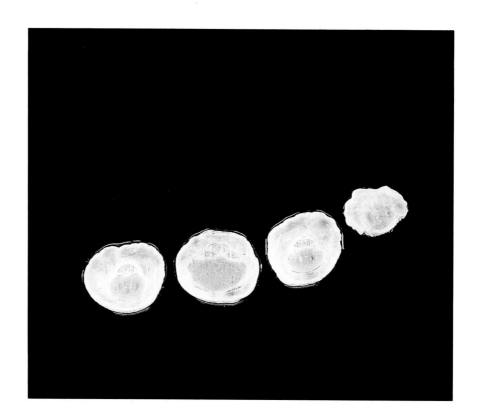

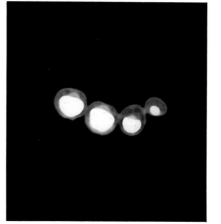

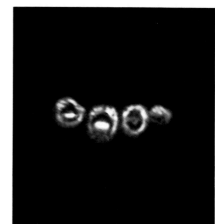

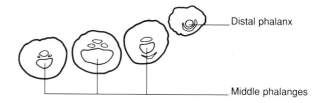

Distal phalanx

Middle phalanges

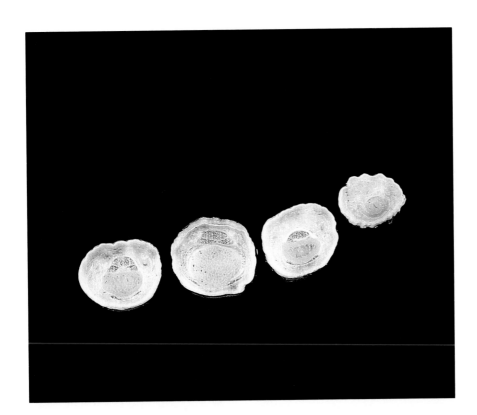

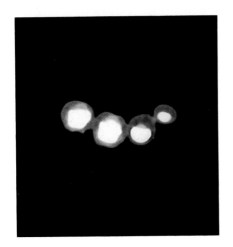

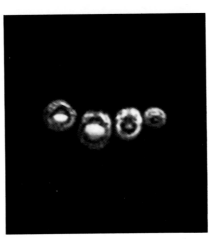

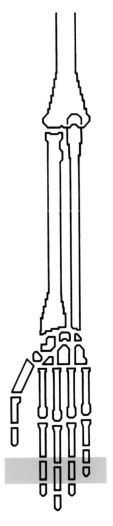

figure 18

figure 19

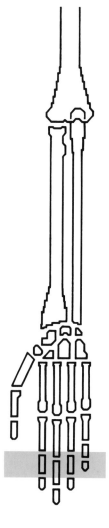

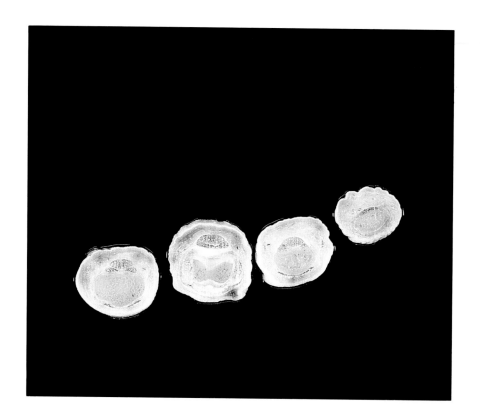

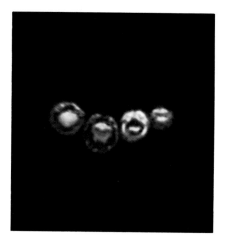

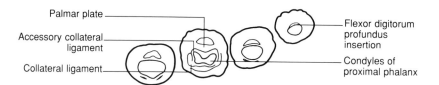

Palmar plate

Accessory collateral ligament

Collateral ligament

Flexor digitorum profundus insertion

Condyles of proximal phalanx

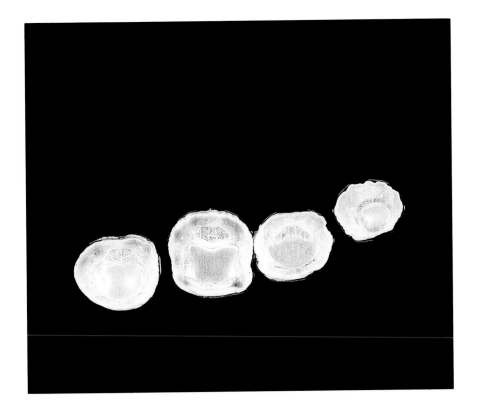

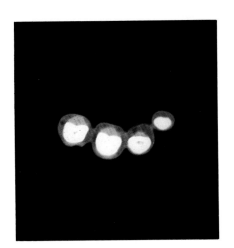

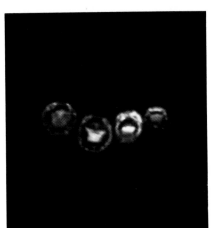

figure 20

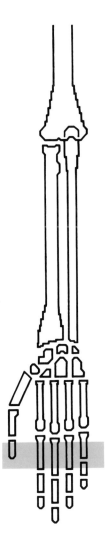

figure 21

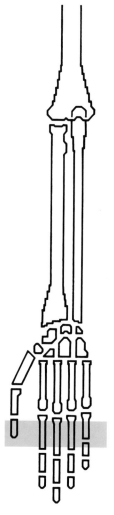

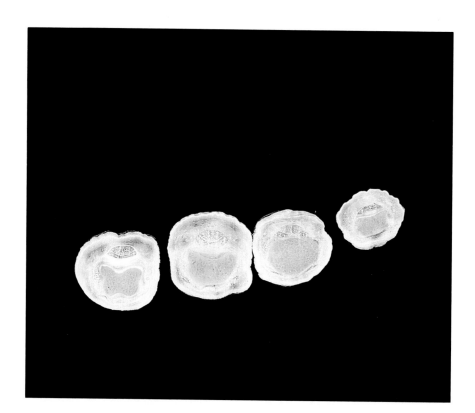

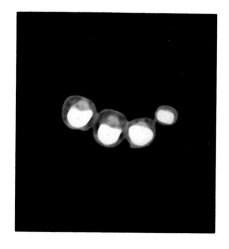

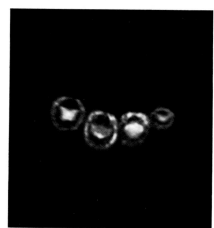

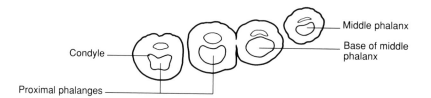

Condyle

Proximal phalanges

Middle phalanx

Base of middle phalanx

figure 22

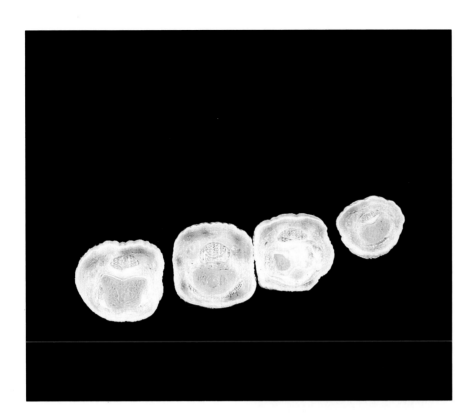

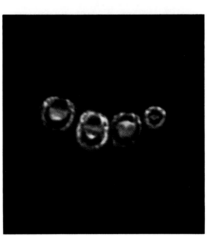

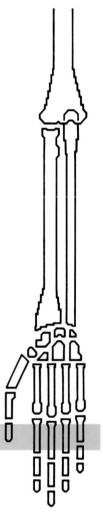

figure 23

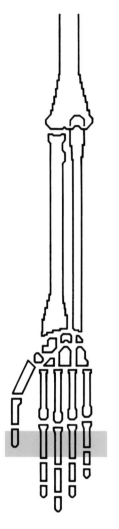

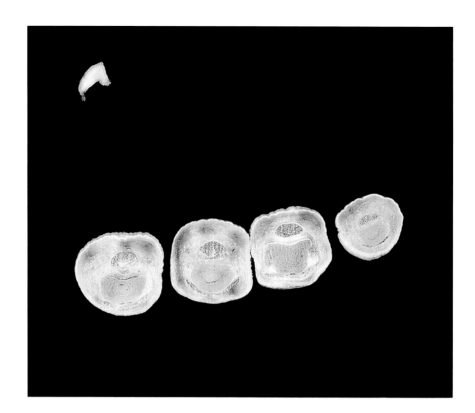

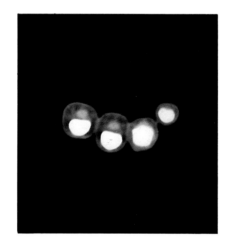

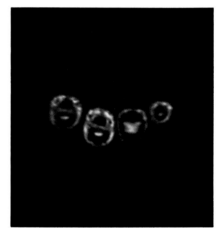

Tip of thumb

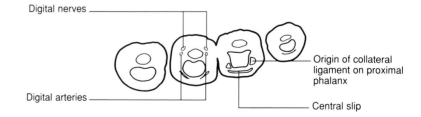

Digital nerves

Digital arteries

Origin of collateral
ligament on proximal
phalanx

Central slip

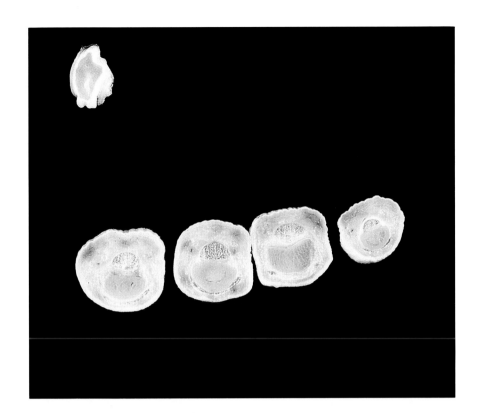

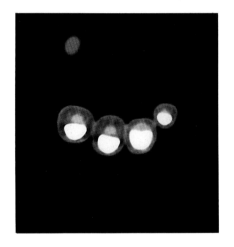

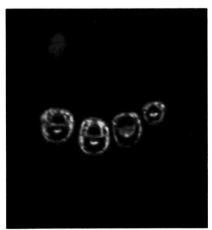

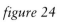

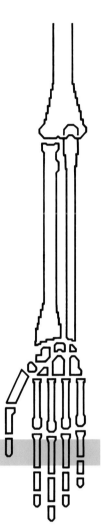

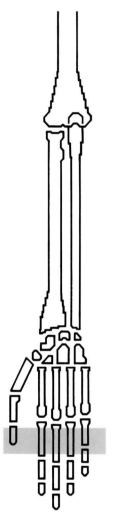

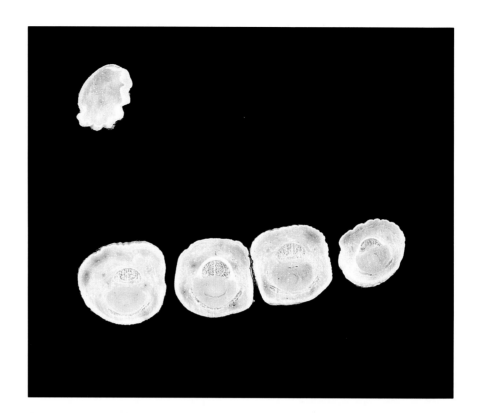

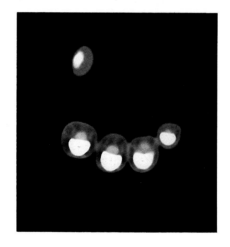

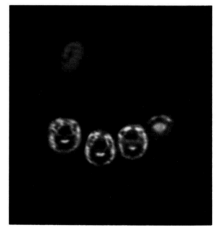

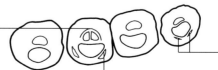

figure 25

Annular pulley enclosing profundus tendon passing through chiasm of superficialis tendon

Conjoined tendons

Lateral band

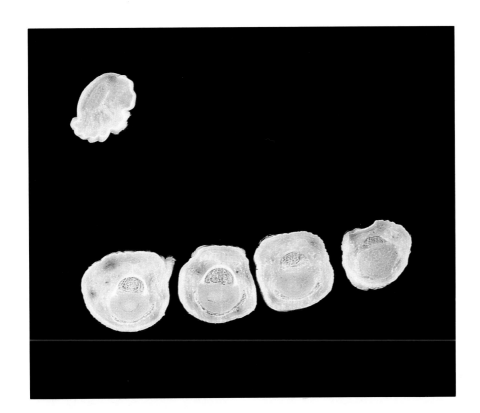

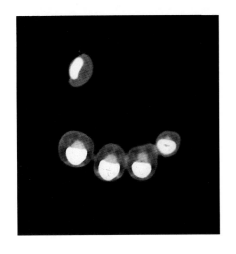

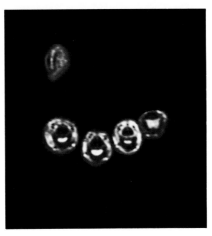

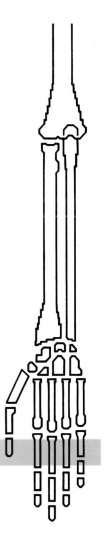

figure 26

figure 27

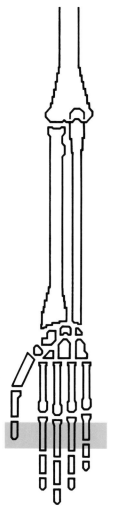

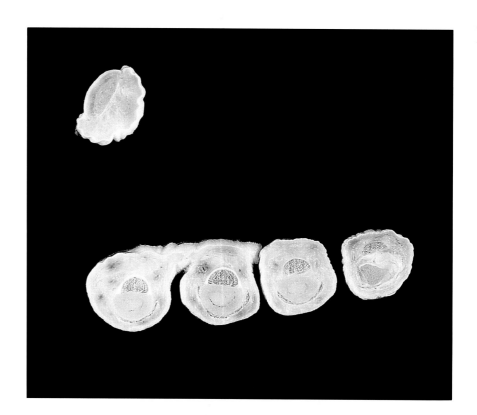

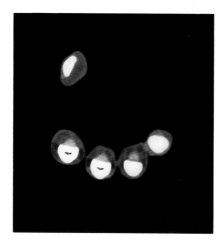
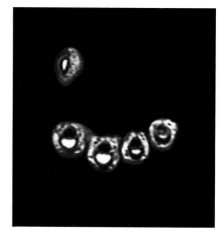

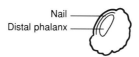

Nail
Distal phalanx

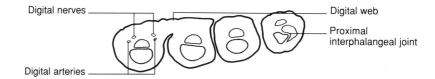

Digital nerves

Digital web

Proximal
interphalangeal joint

Digital arteries

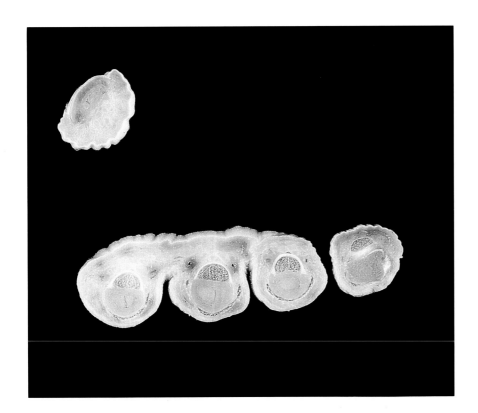

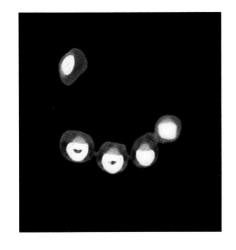
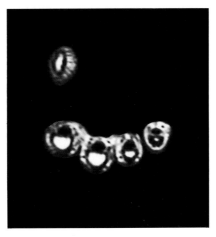

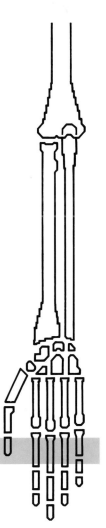

figure 28

figure 29

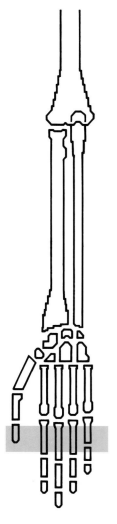

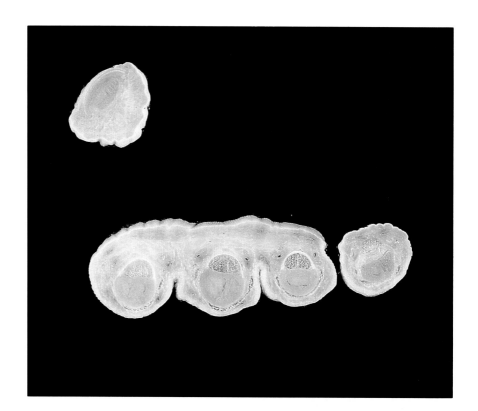

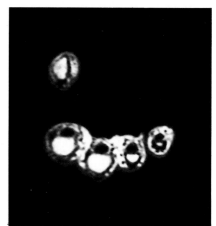

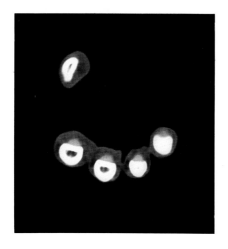

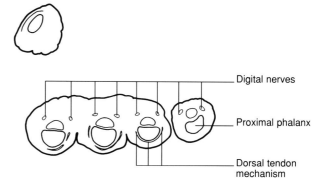

Digital nerves

Proximal phalanx

Dorsal tendon
mechanism

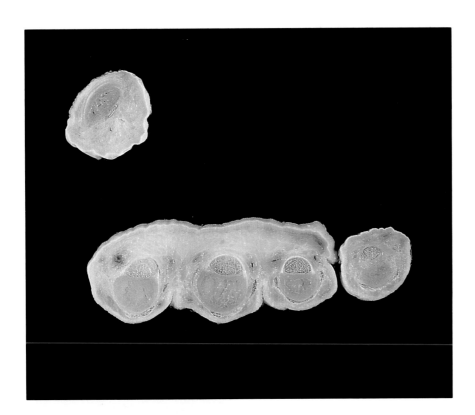

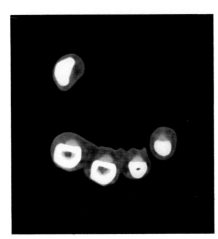

figure 30

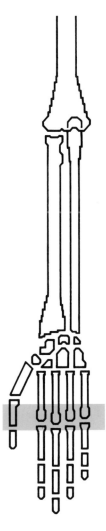

figure 31

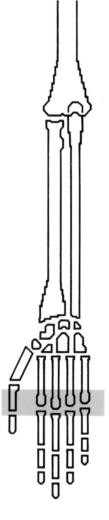

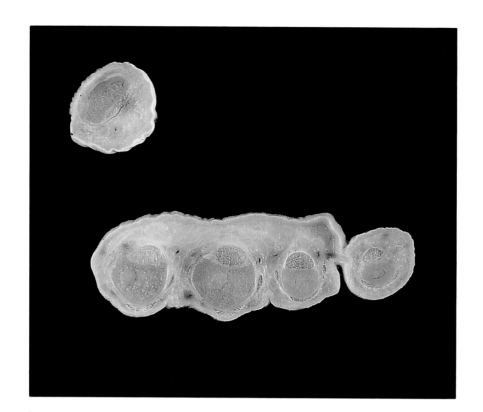

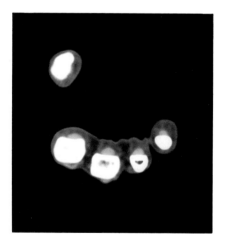

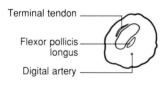

Terminal tendon

Flexor pollicis longus

Digital artery

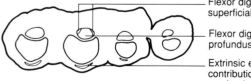

Flexor digitorum superficialis

Flexor digitorum profundus

Extrinsic extensor contribution to dorsal mechanism

figure 32

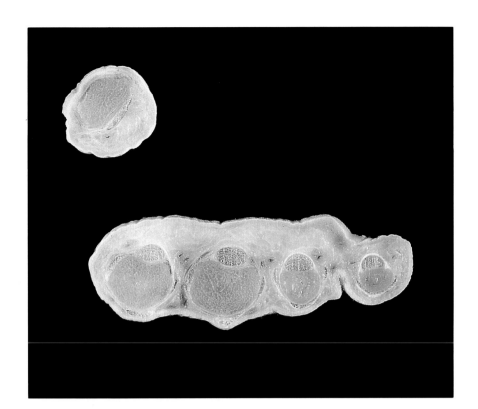

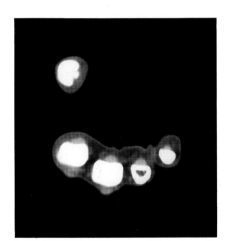

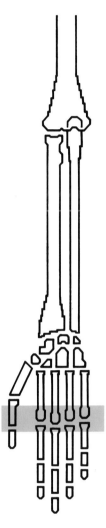

figure 33

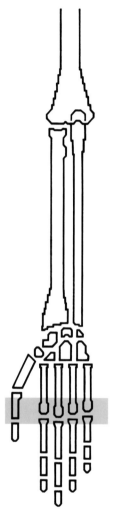

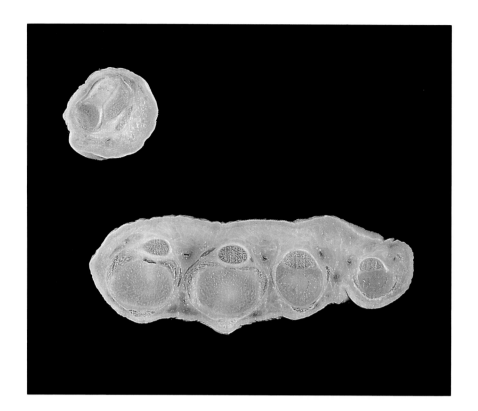

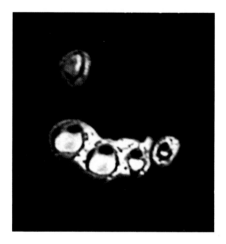

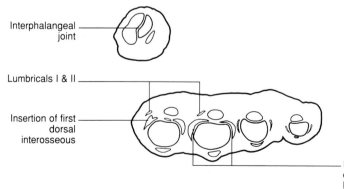

Interphalangeal joint

Lumbricals I & II

Insertion of first dorsal interosseous

Insertion of collateral ligaments on base of proximal phalanx

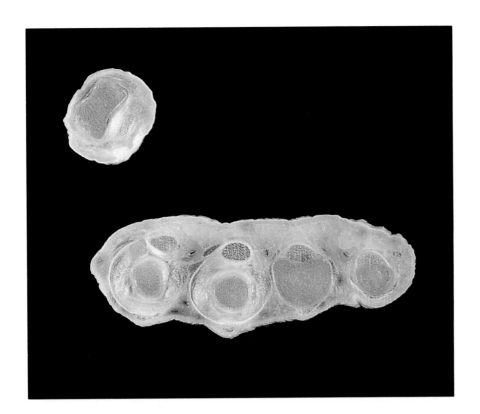

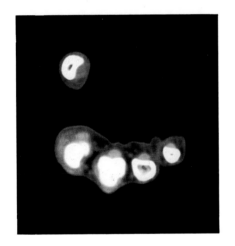
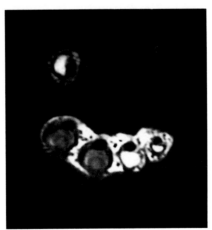

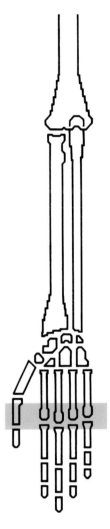

figure 34

figure 35

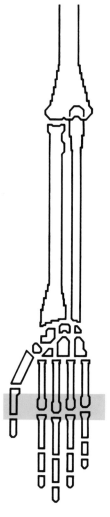

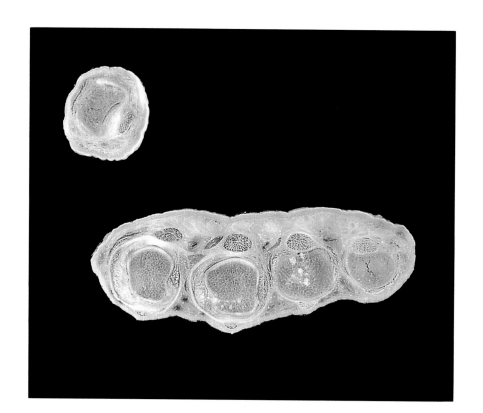

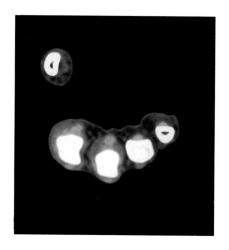

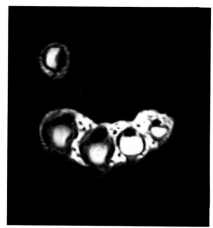

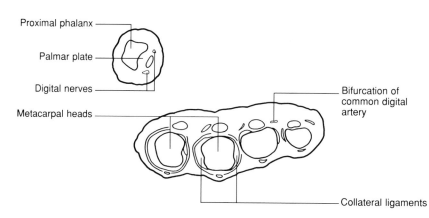

Proximal phalanx

Palmar plate

Digital nerves

Metacarpal heads

Bifurcation of
common digital
artery

Collateral ligaments

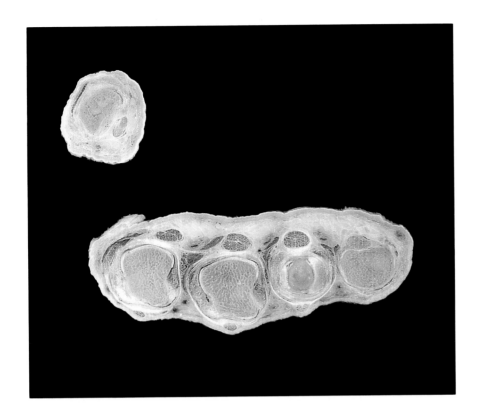

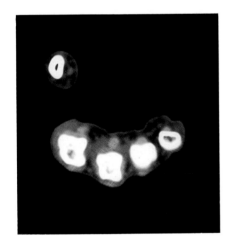

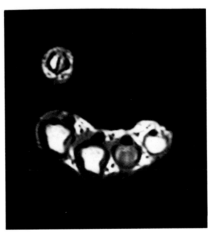

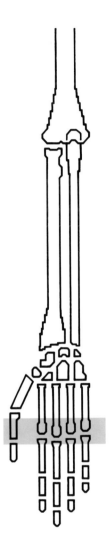

figure 36

figure 37

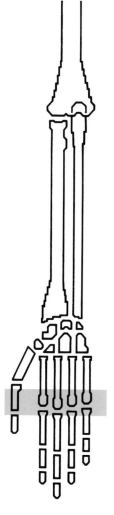

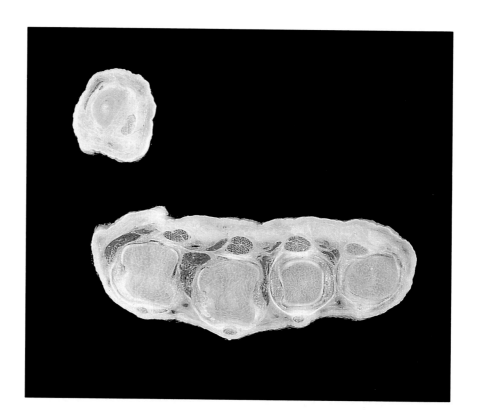

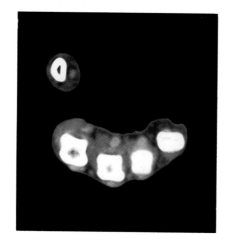

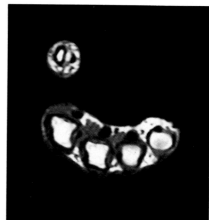

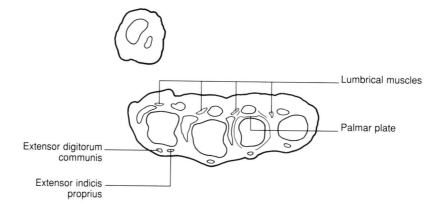

Lumbrical muscles

Palmar plate

Extensor digitorum communis

Extensor indicis proprius

figure 38

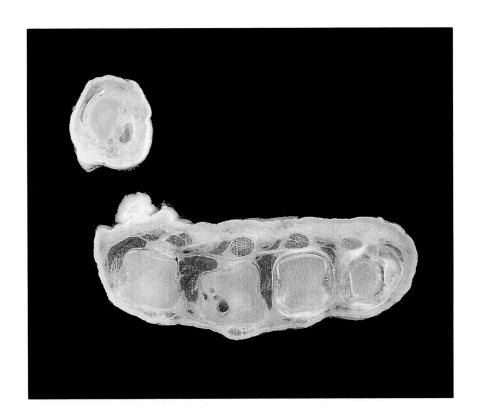

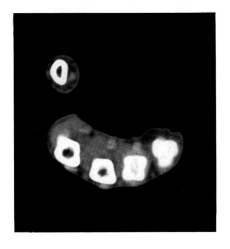

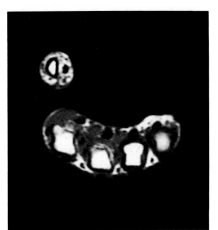

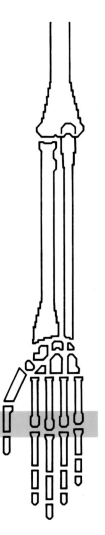

figure 39

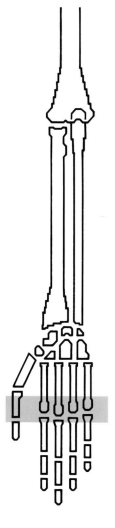

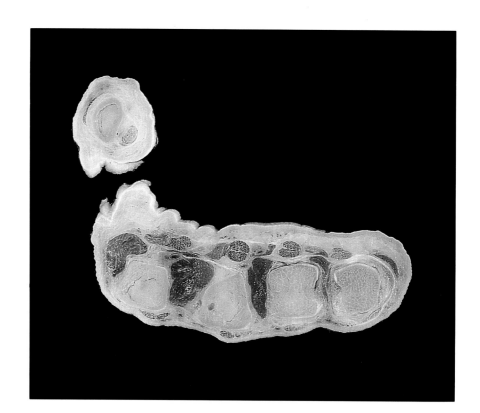

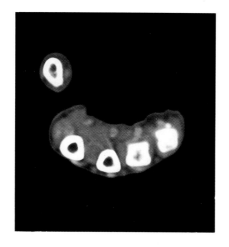

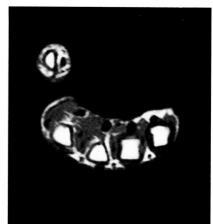

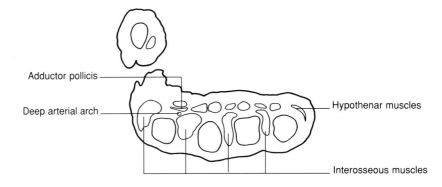

Adductor pollicis

Deep arterial arch

Hypothenar muscles

Interosseous muscles

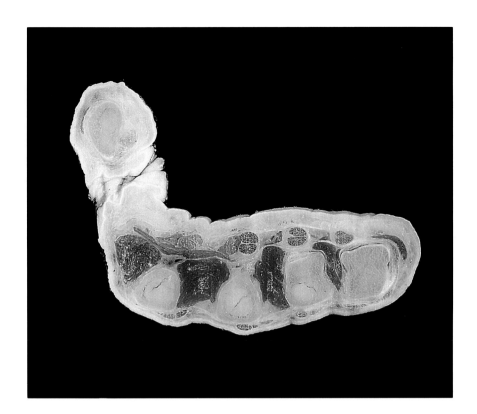

figure 40

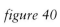

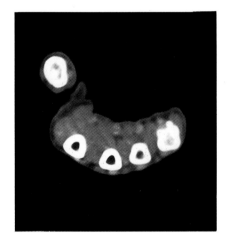

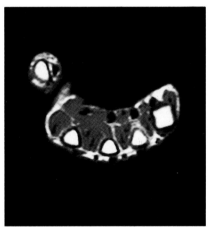

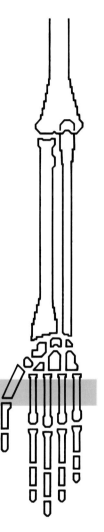

figure 41

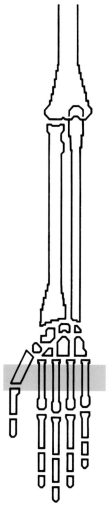

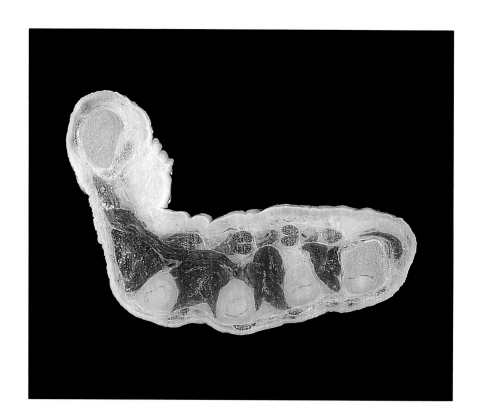

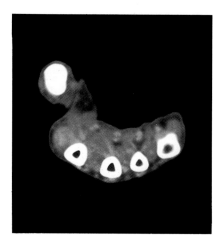
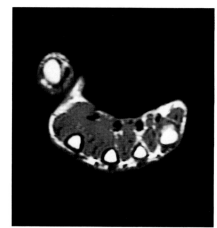

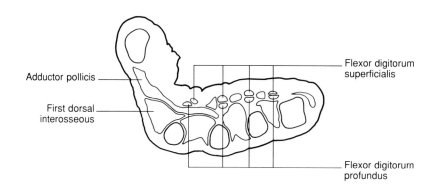

Adductor pollicis

First dorsal
interosseous

Flexor digitorum
superficialis

Flexor digitorum
profundus

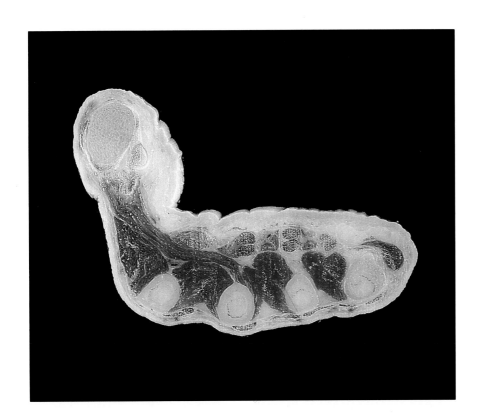

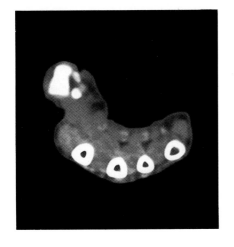

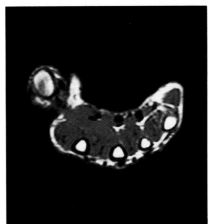

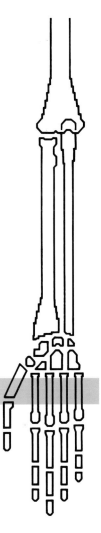

figure 42

figure 43

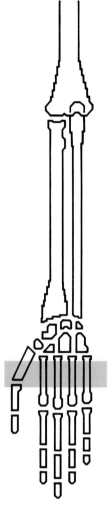

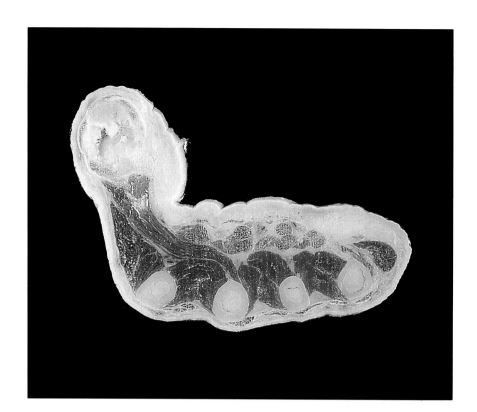

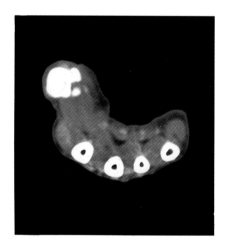
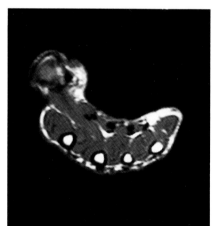

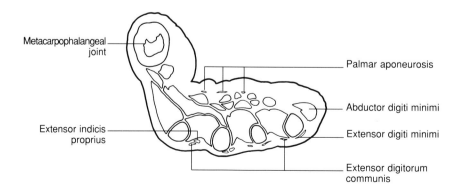

Metacarpophalangeal joint

Palmar aponeurosis

Abductor digiti minimi

Extensor indicis proprius

Extensor digiti minimi

Extensor digitorum communis

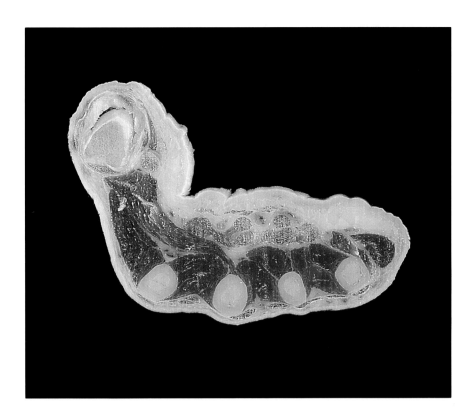

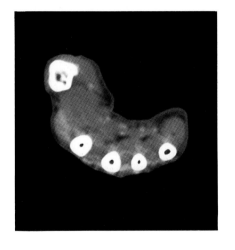

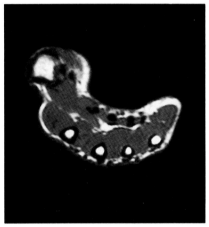

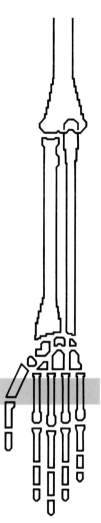

figure 44

figure 45

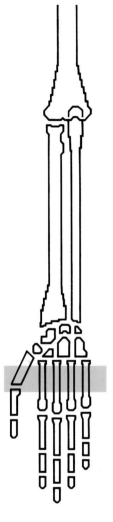

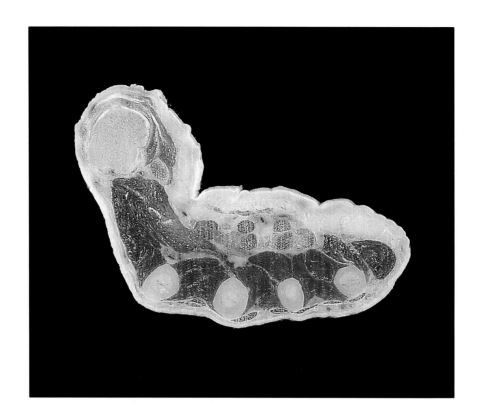

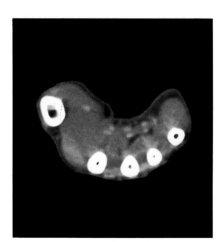

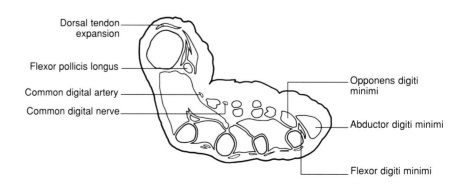

Dorsal tendon expansion

Flexor pollicis longus

Common digital artery

Common digital nerve

Opponens digiti minimi

Abductor digiti minimi

Flexor digiti minimi

figure 46

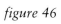

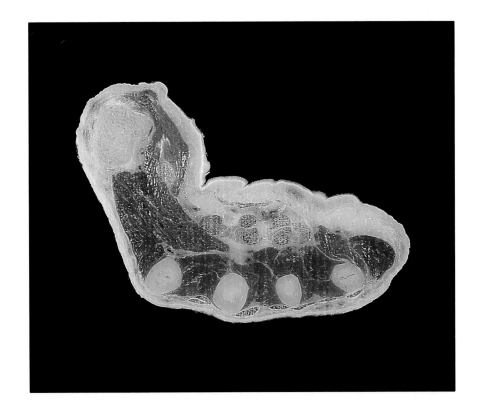

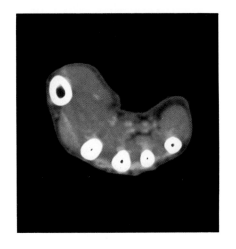

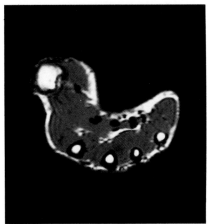

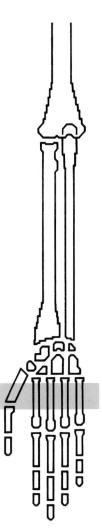

figure 47

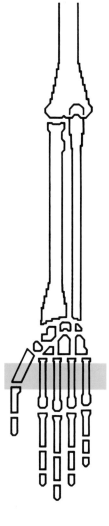

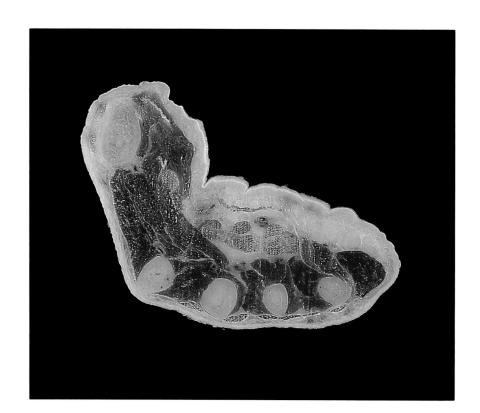

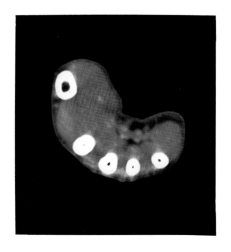

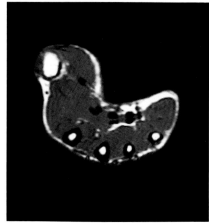

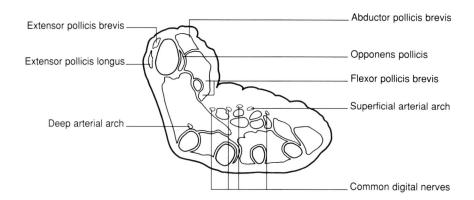

Extensor pollicis brevis

Extensor pollicis longus

Deep arterial arch

Abductor pollicis brevis

Opponens pollicis

Flexor pollicis brevis

Superficial arterial arch

Common digital nerves

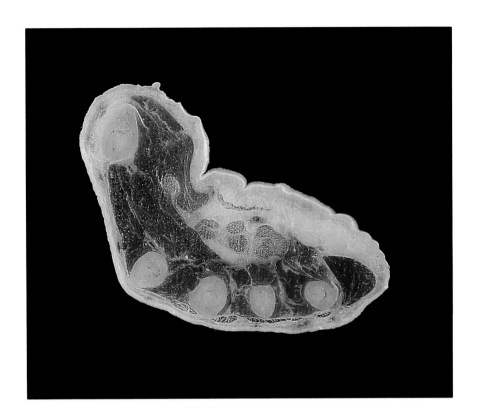

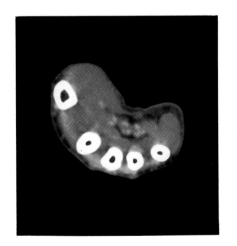 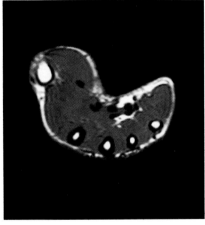

figure 48

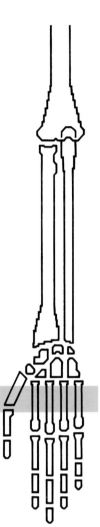

figure 49

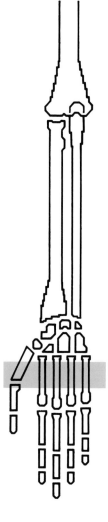

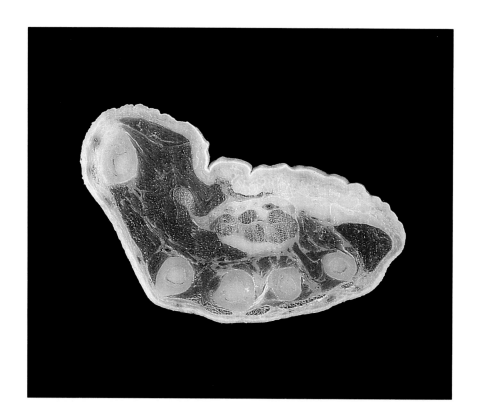

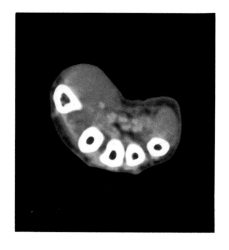

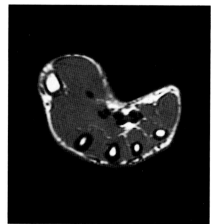

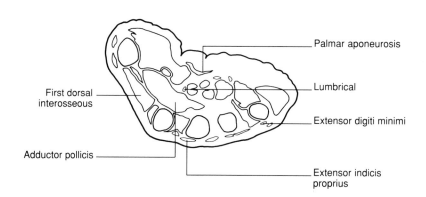

First dorsal interosseous

Adductor pollicis

Palmar aponeurosis

Lumbrical

Extensor digiti minimi

Extensor indicis proprius

figure 50

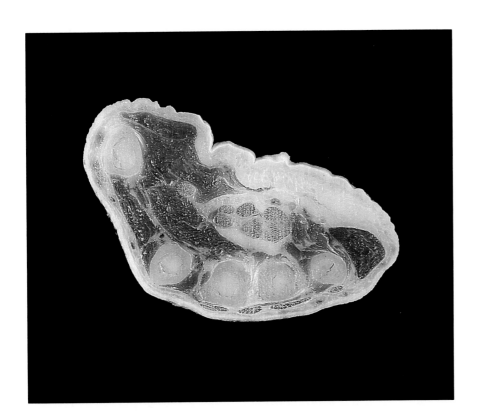

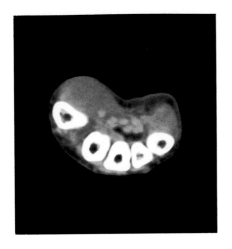

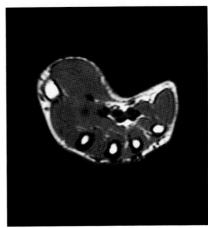

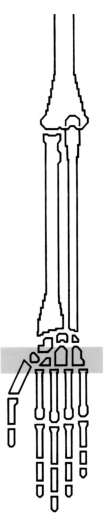

figure 51

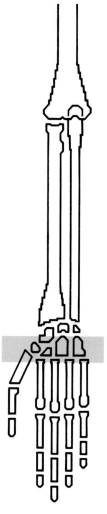

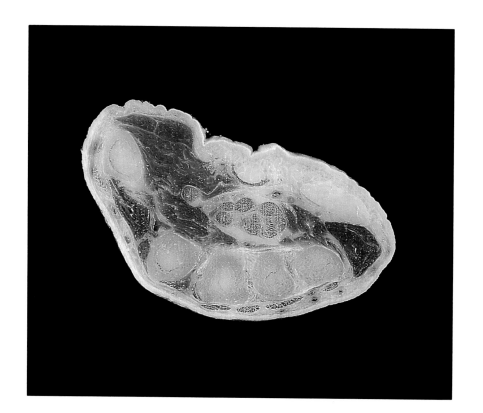

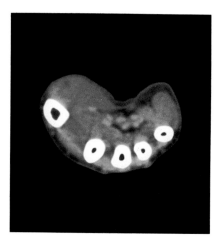

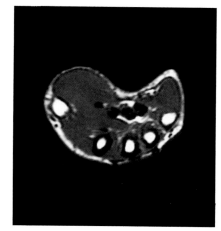

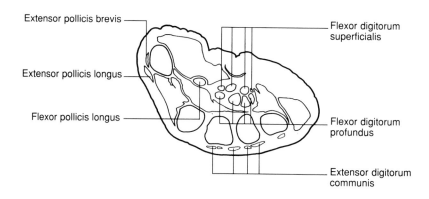

Extensor pollicis brevis — | — Flexor digitorum superficialis

Extensor pollicis longus — | — Flexor digitorum profundus

Flexor pollicis longus — | — Extensor digitorum communis

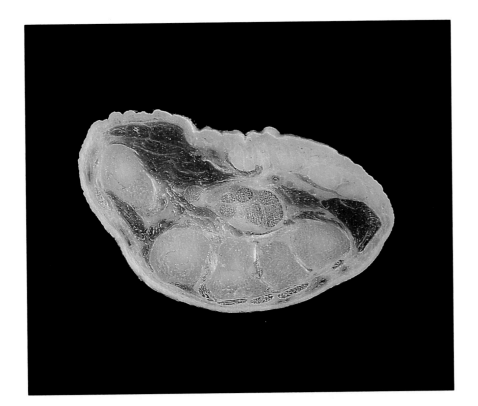

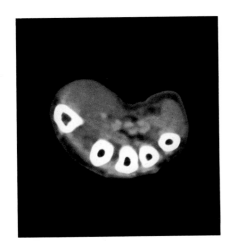 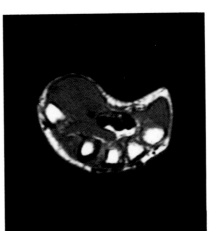

figure 52

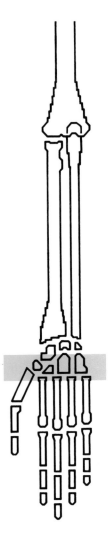

figure 53

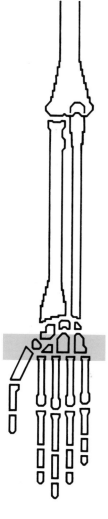

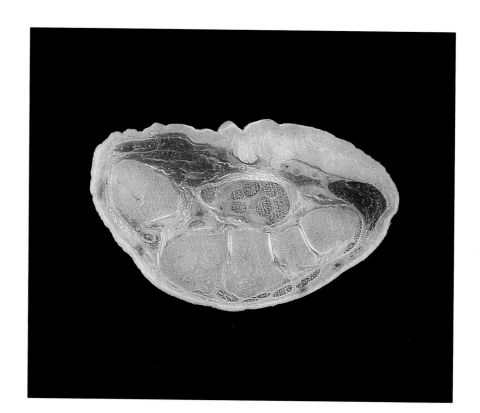

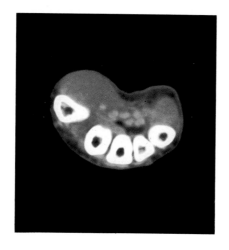

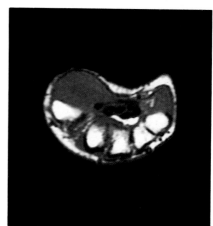

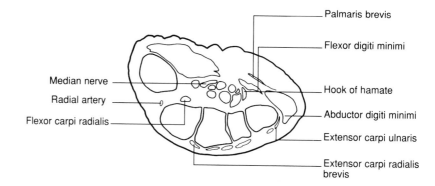

Palmaris brevis

Flexor digiti minimi

Median nerve

Hook of hamate

Radial artery

Abductor digiti minimi

Flexor carpi radialis

Extensor carpi ulnaris

Extensor carpi radialis brevis

figure 54

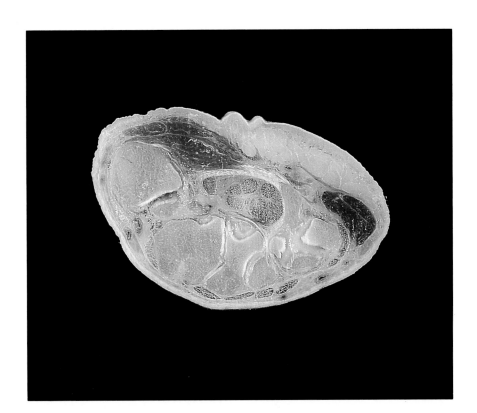

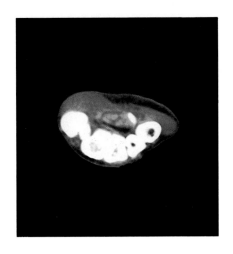
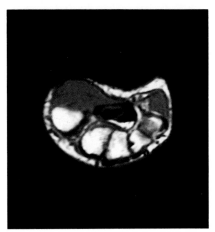

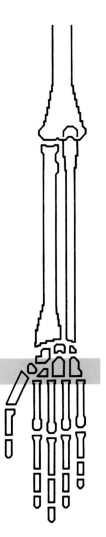

figure 55

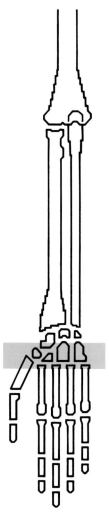

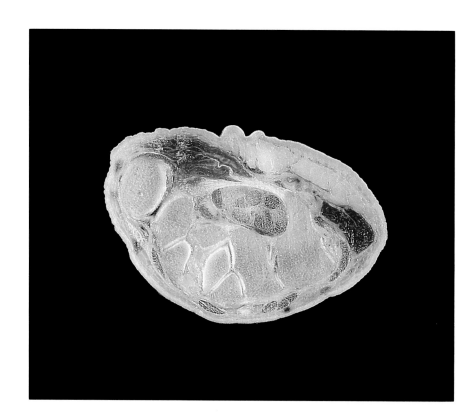

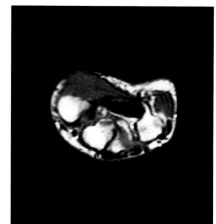

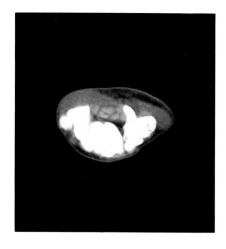

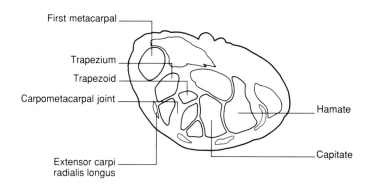

First metacarpal

Trapezium

Trapezoid

Carpometacarpal joint

Hamate

Capitate

Extensor carpi
radialis longus

figure 56

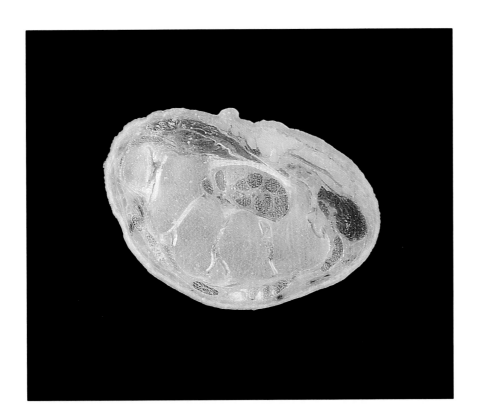

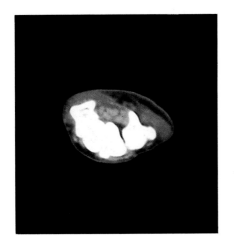

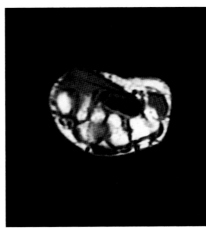

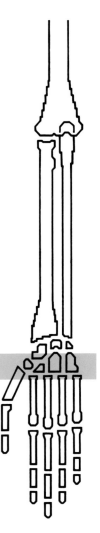

figure 57

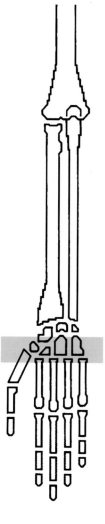

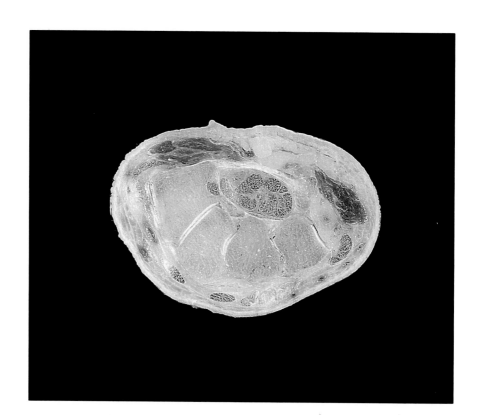

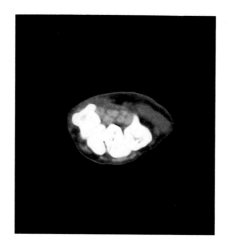

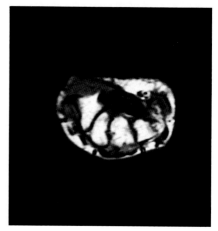

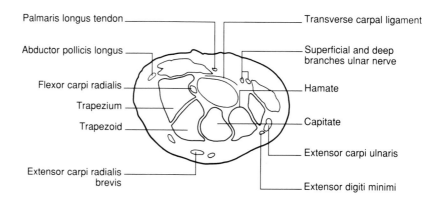

Palmaris longus tendon

Abductor pollicis longus

Flexor carpi radialis

Trapezium

Trapezoid

Extensor carpi radialis brevis

Transverse carpal ligament

Superficial and deep branches ulnar nerve

Hamate

Capitate

Extensor carpi ulnaris

Extensor digiti minimi

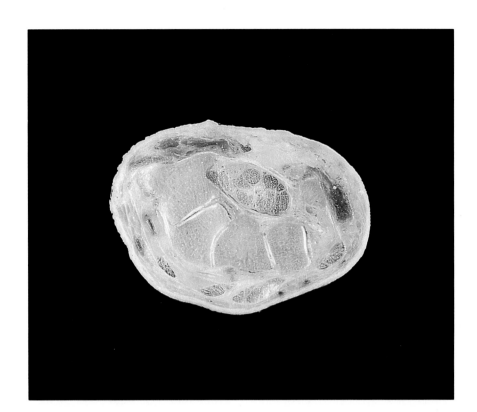

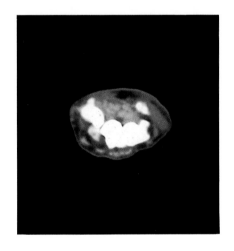
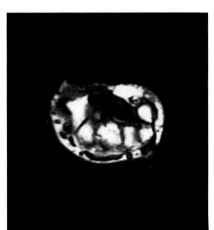

figure 58

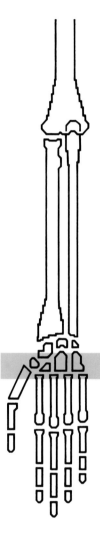

figure 59

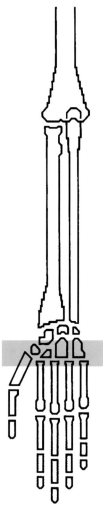

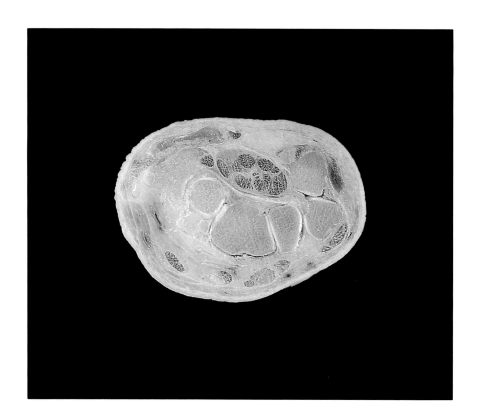

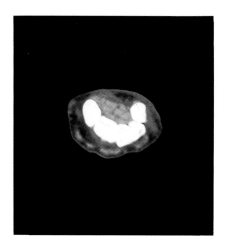

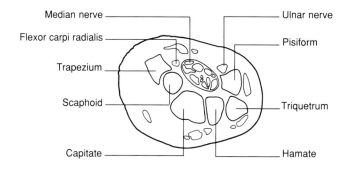

Median nerve

Flexor carpi radialis

Trapezium

Scaphoid

Capitate

Ulnar nerve

Pisiform

Triquetrum

Hamate

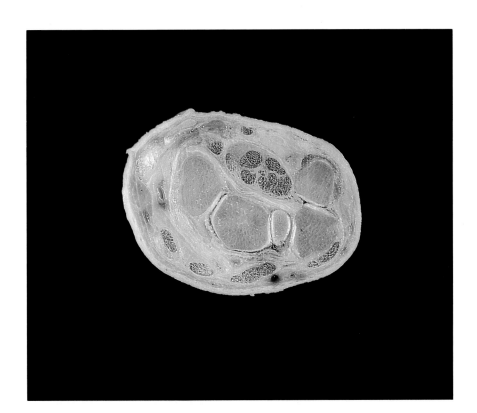

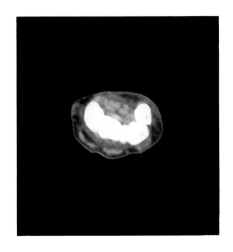

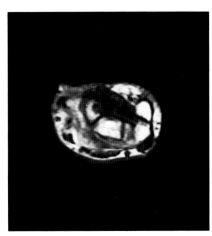

figure 60

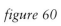

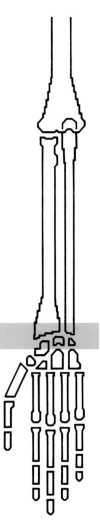

figure 61

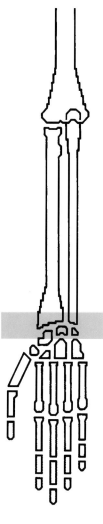

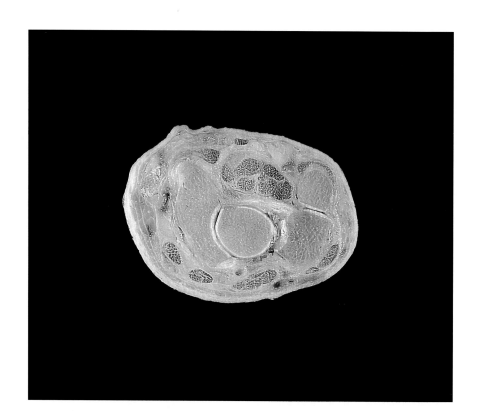

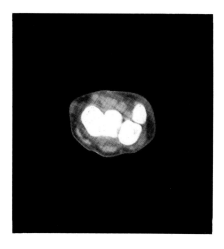

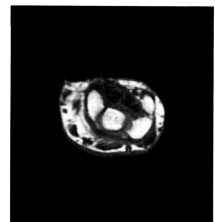

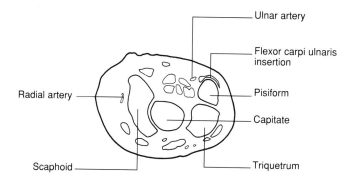

Ulnar artery

Flexor carpi ulnaris insertion

Pisiform

Radial artery

Capitate

Scaphoid

Triquetrum

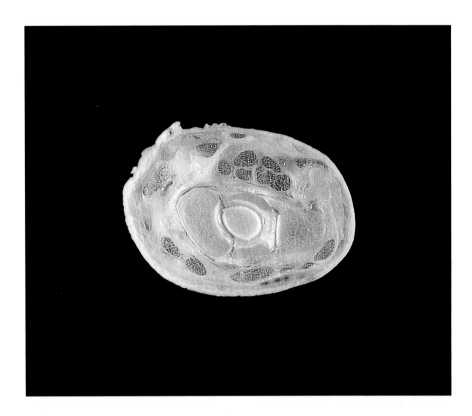

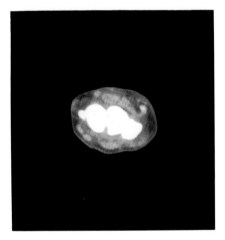 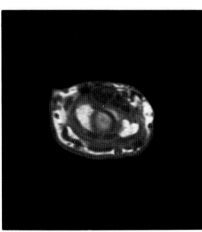

figure 62

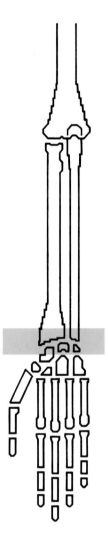

figure 63

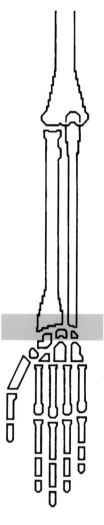

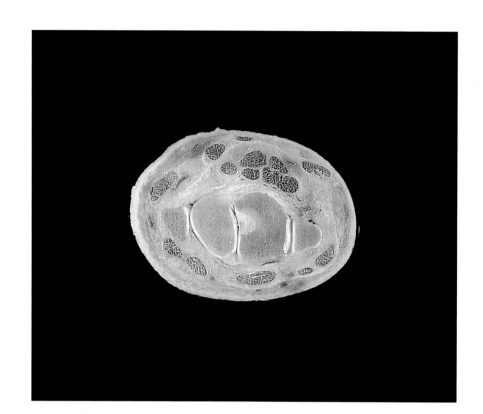

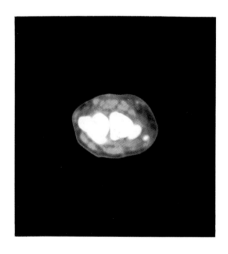
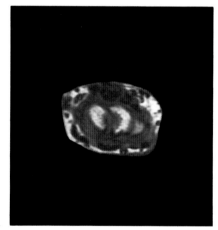

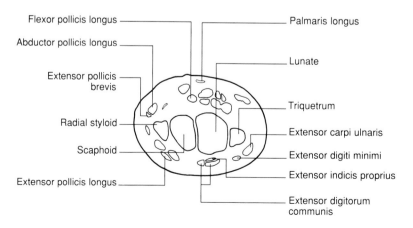

Flexor pollicis longus

Abductor pollicis longus

Extensor pollicis brevis

Radial styloid

Scaphoid

Extensor pollicis longus

Palmaris longus

Lunate

Triquetrum

Extensor carpi ulnaris

Extensor digiti minimi

Extensor indicis proprius

Extensor digitorum communis

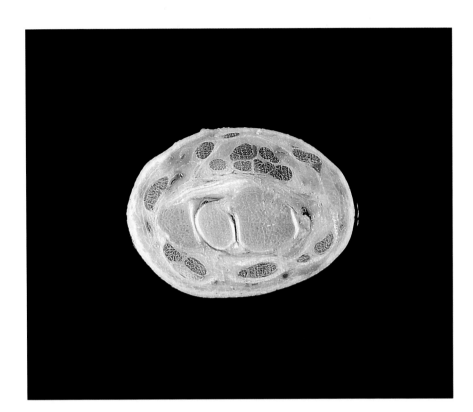

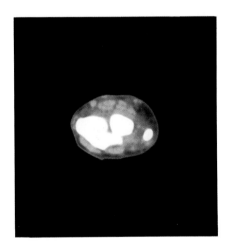

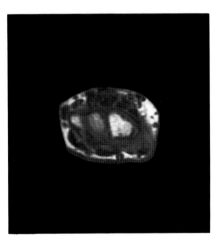

figure 64

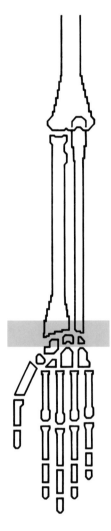

figure 65

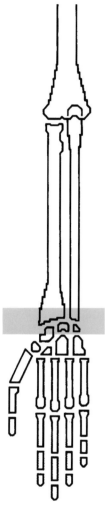

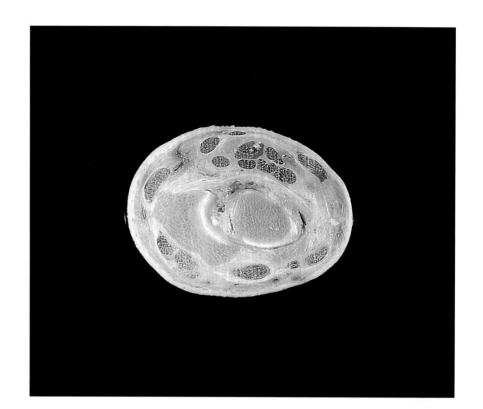

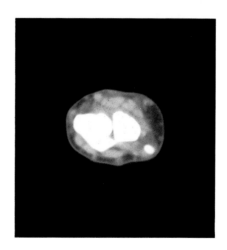

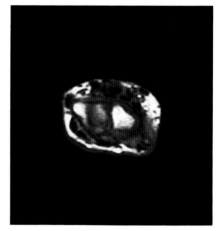

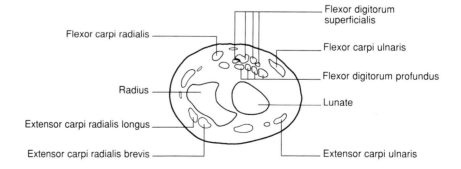

Flexor carpi radialis

Radius

Extensor carpi radialis longus

Extensor carpi radialis brevis

Flexor digitorum
superficialis

Flexor carpi ulnaris

Flexor digitorum profundus

Lunate

Extensor carpi ulnaris

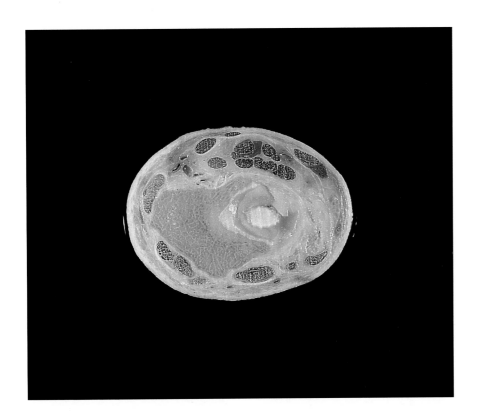

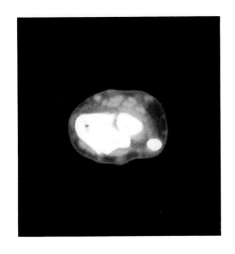

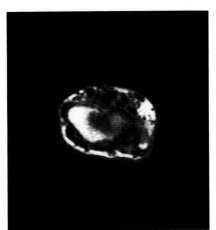

figure 66

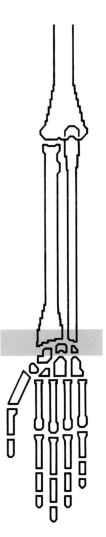

figure 67

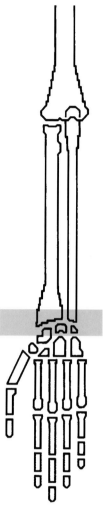

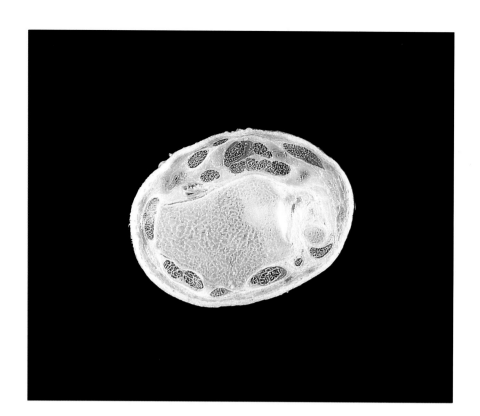

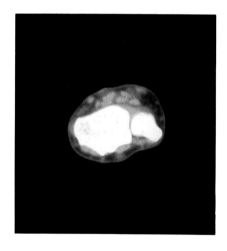

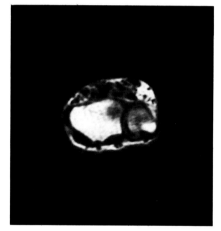

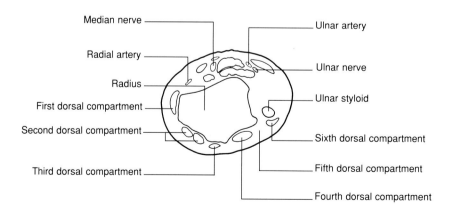

Median nerve

Radial artery

Radius

First dorsal compartment

Second dorsal compartment

Third dorsal compartment

Ulnar artery

Ulnar nerve

Ulnar styloid

Sixth dorsal compartment

Fifth dorsal compartment

Fourth dorsal compartment

figure 68

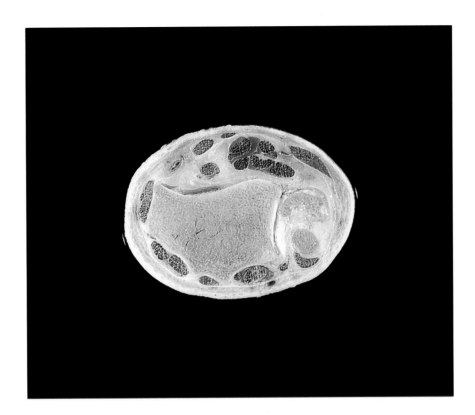

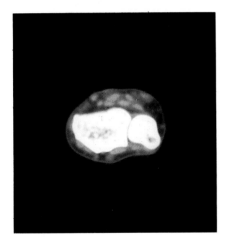

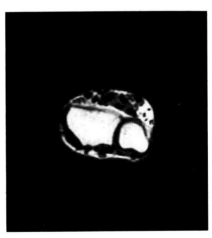

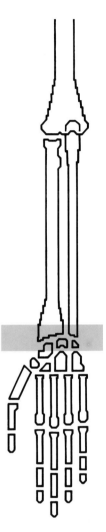

figure 69

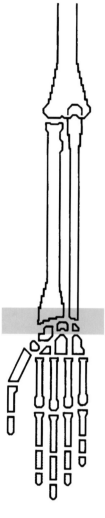

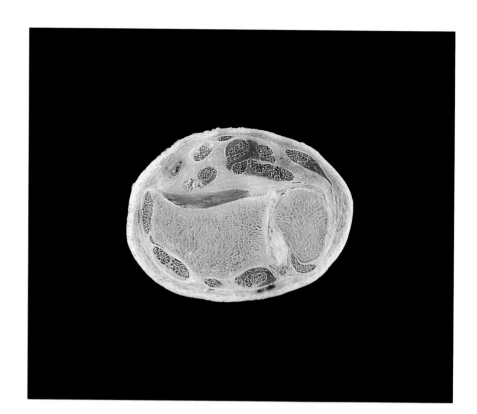

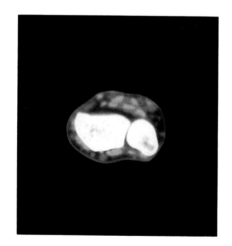

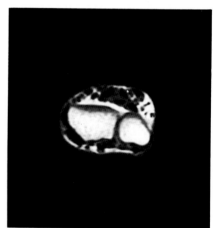

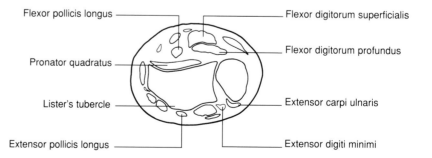

Flexor pollicis longus

Pronator quadratus

Lister's tubercle

Extensor pollicis longus

Flexor digitorum superficialis

Flexor digitorum profundus

Extensor carpi ulnaris

Extensor digiti minimi

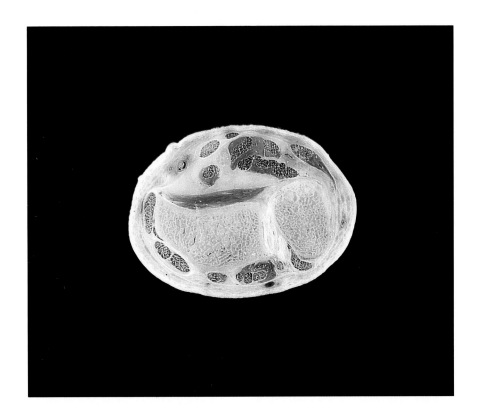

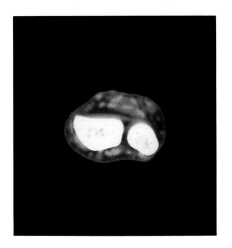

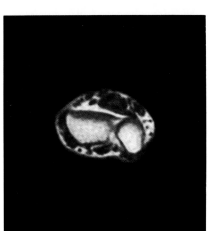

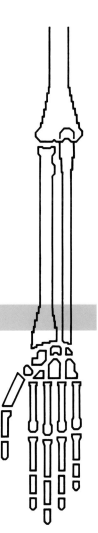

figure 70

figure 71

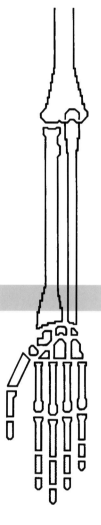

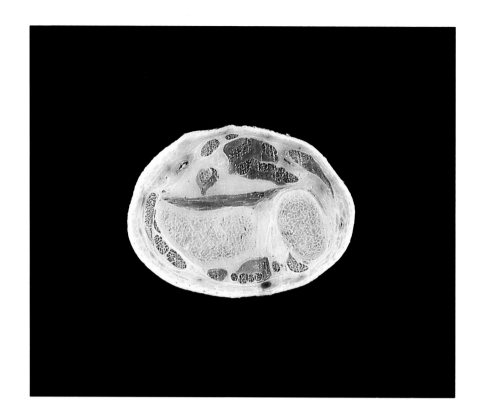

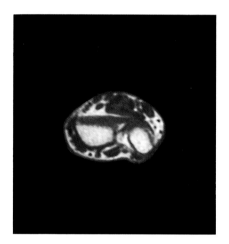

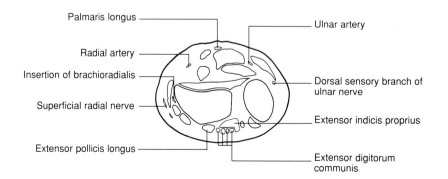

Palmaris longus

Radial artery

Insertion of brachioradialis

Superficial radial nerve

Extensor pollicis longus

Ulnar artery

Dorsal sensory branch of ulnar nerve

Extensor indicis proprius

Extensor digitorum communis

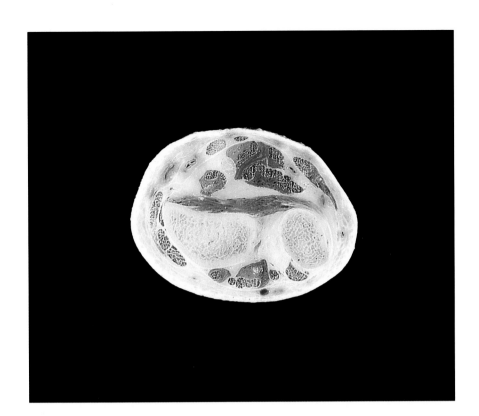

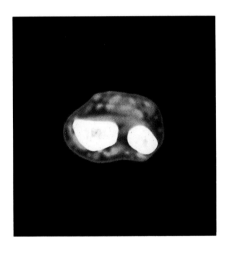

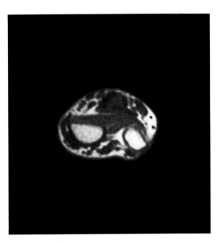

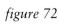

figure 72

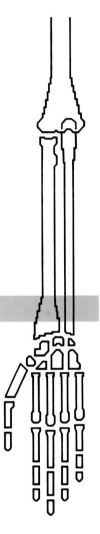

figure 73

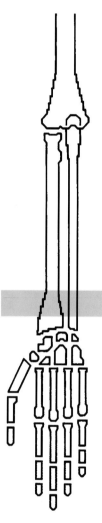

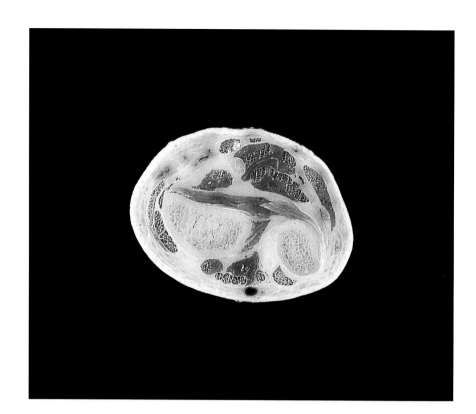

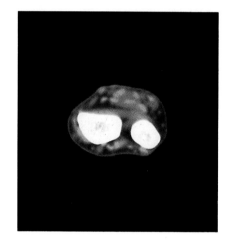

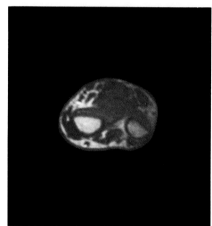

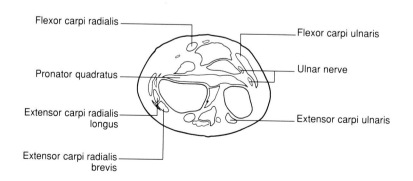

Flexor carpi radialis

Pronator quadratus

Extensor carpi radialis
longus

Extensor carpi radialis
brevis

Flexor carpi ulnaris

Ulnar nerve

Extensor carpi ulnaris

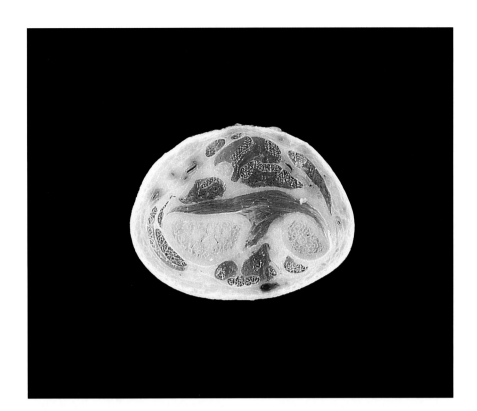

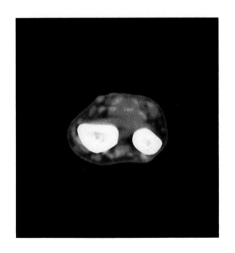

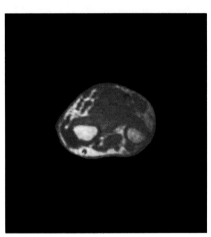

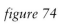

figure 74

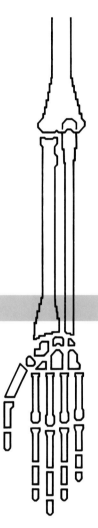

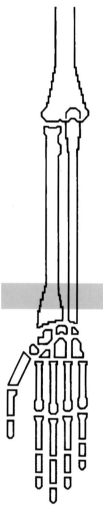

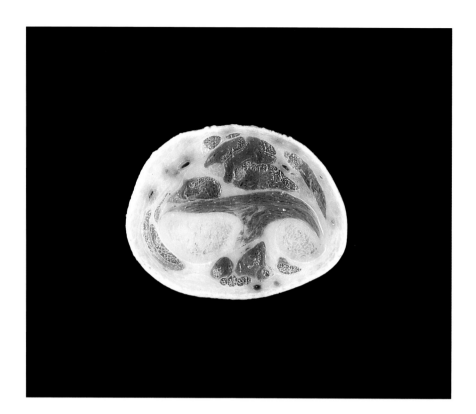

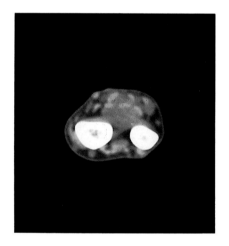

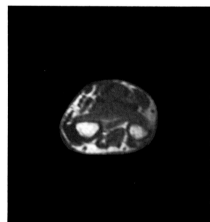

figure 75

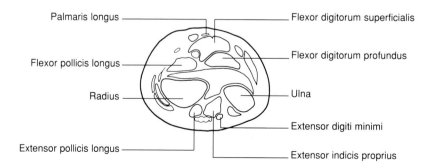

Palmaris longus — Flexor digitorum superficialis

Flexor pollicis longus — Flexor digitorum profundus

Radius — Ulna

Extensor pollicis longus — Extensor digiti minimi

Extensor indicis proprius

figure 76

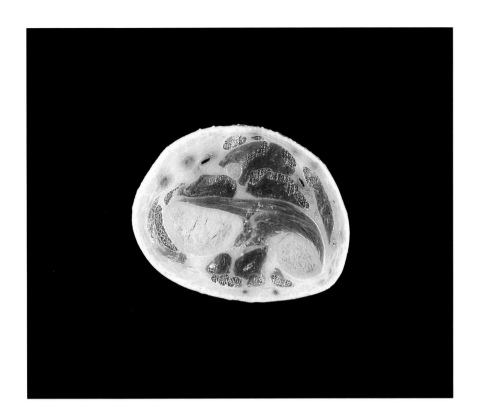

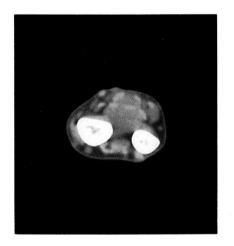

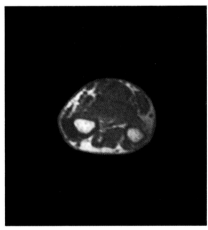

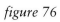

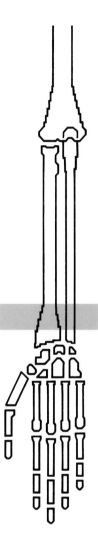

figure 77

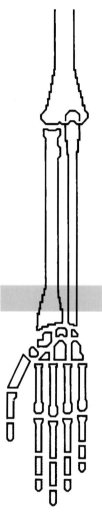

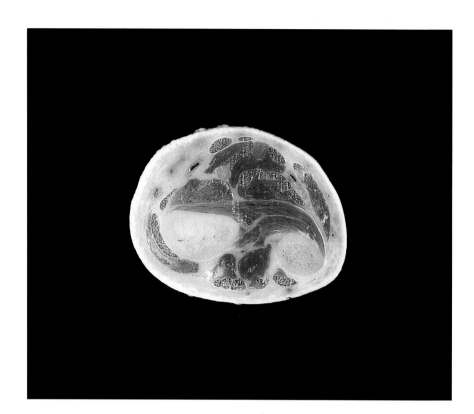

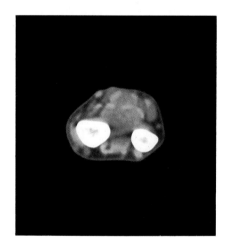

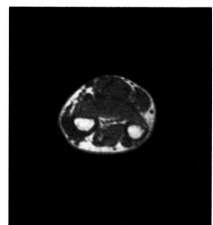

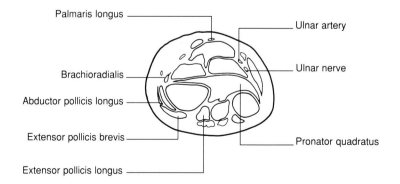

Palmaris longus

Brachioradialis

Abductor pollicis longus

Extensor pollicis brevis

Extensor pollicis longus

Ulnar artery

Ulnar nerve

Pronator quadratus

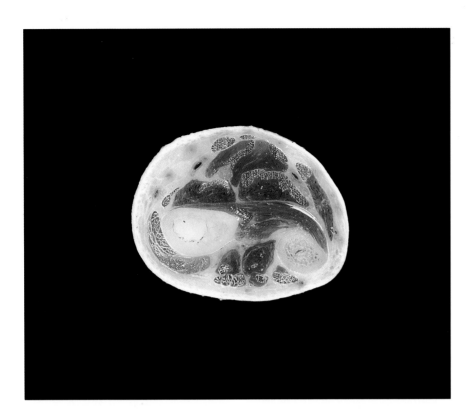

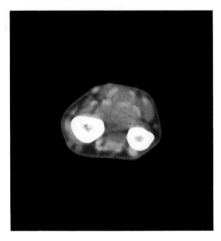

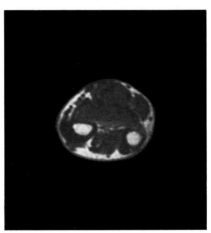

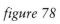

figure 78

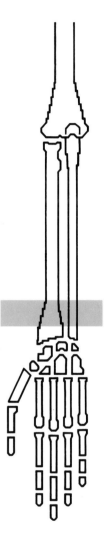

figure 79

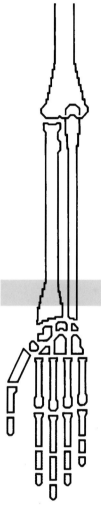

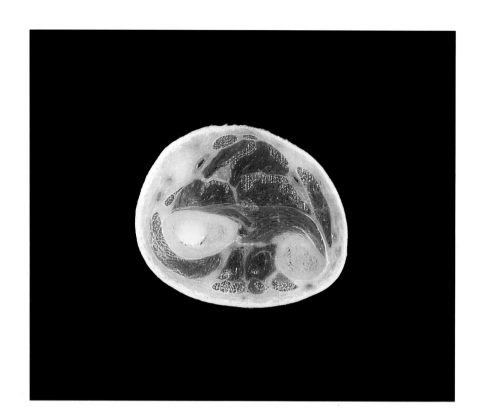

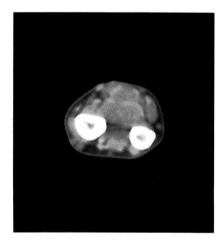

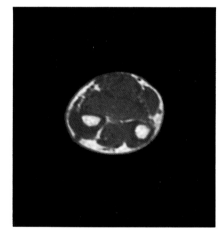

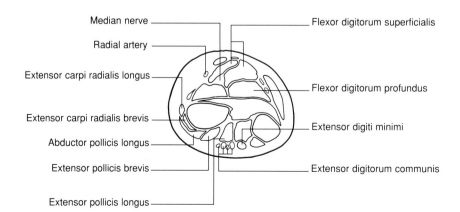

Median nerve	Flexor digitorum superficialis
Radial artery	
Extensor carpi radialis longus	Flexor digitorum profundus
Extensor carpi radialis brevis	Extensor digiti minimi
Abductor pollicis longus	
Extensor pollicis brevis	Extensor digitorum communis
Extensor pollicis longus	

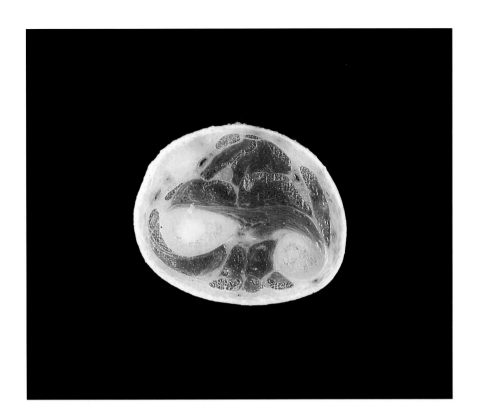

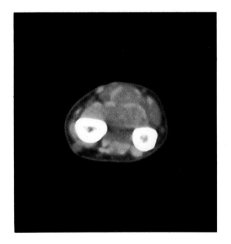

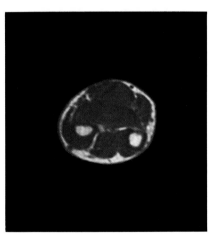

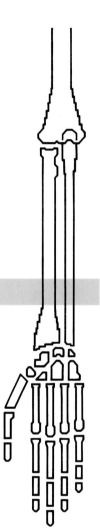

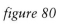 *figure 80*

figure 81

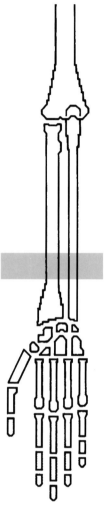

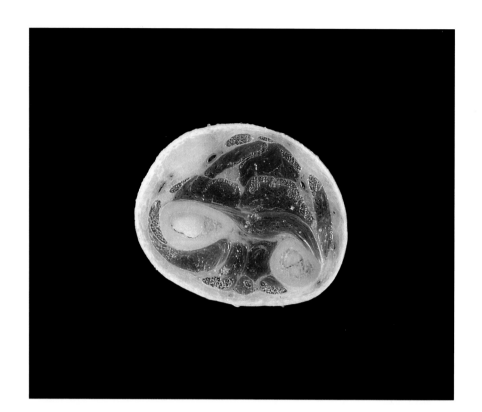

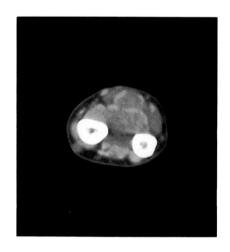

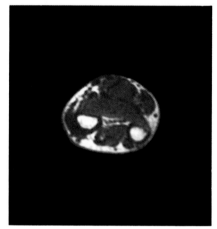

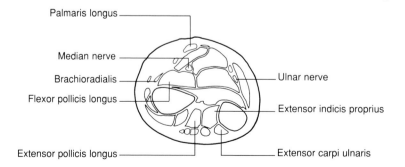

Palmaris longus

Median nerve

Brachioradialis

Flexor pollicis longus

Ulnar nerve

Extensor indicis proprius

Extensor pollicis longus

Extensor carpi ulnaris

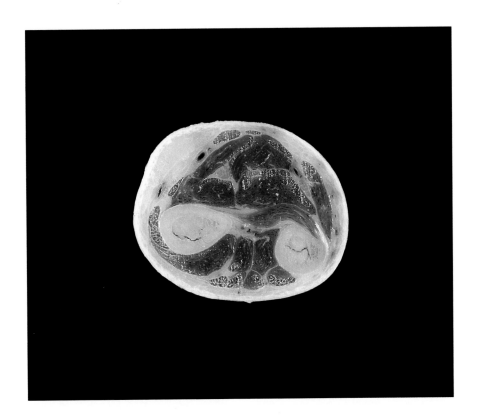

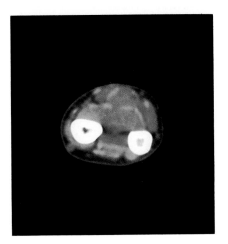

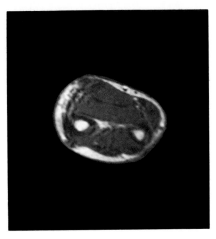

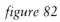
figure 82

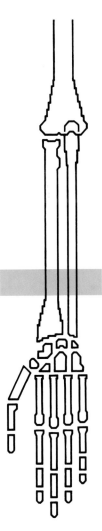

figure 83

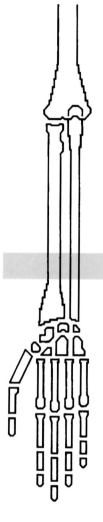

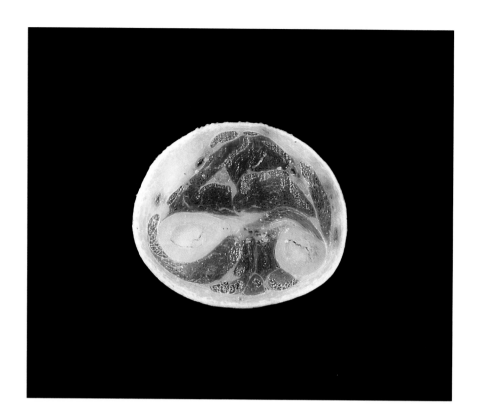

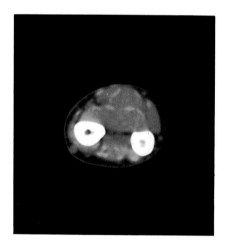

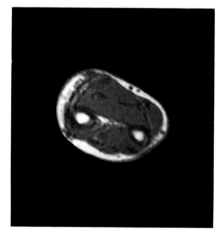

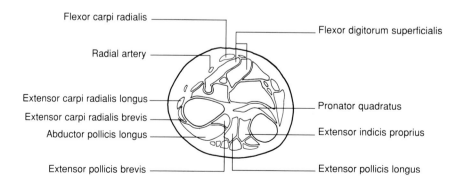

Flexor carpi radialis

Flexor digitorum superficialis

Radial artery

Extensor carpi radialis longus

Extensor carpi radialis brevis

Abductor pollicis longus

Pronator quadratus

Extensor indicis proprius

Extensor pollicis brevis

Extensor pollicis longus

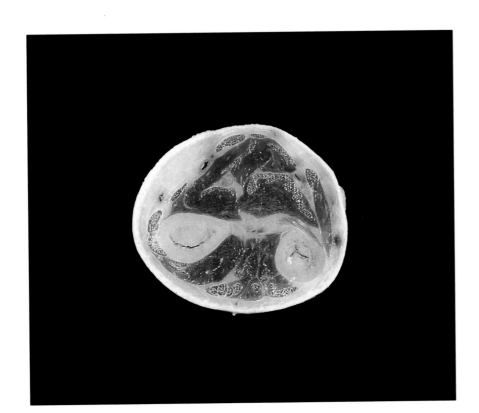

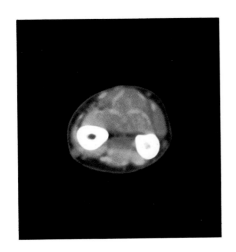

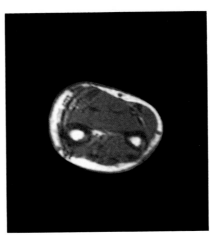

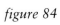

figure 84

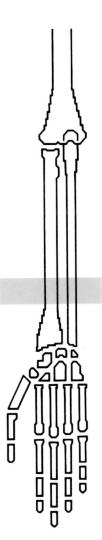

figure 85

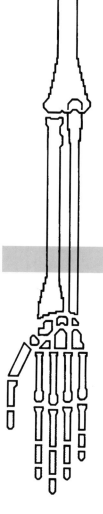

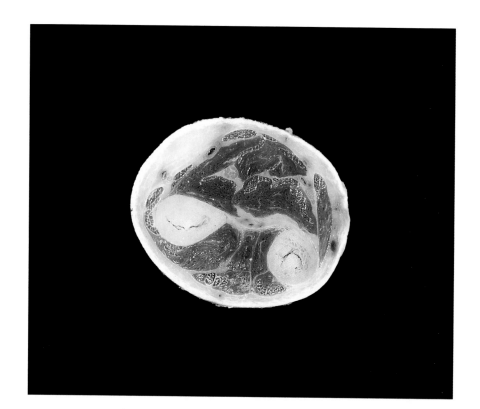

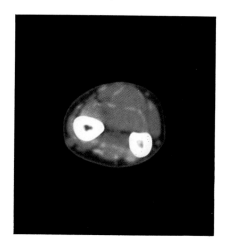

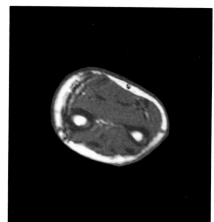

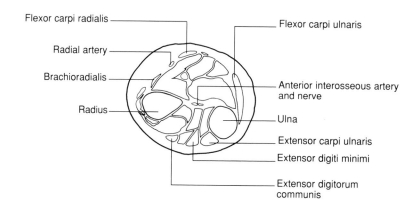

Flexor carpi radialis

Radial artery

Brachioradialis

Radius

Flexor carpi ulnaris

Anterior interosseous artery and nerve

Ulna

Extensor carpi ulnaris

Extensor digiti minimi

Extensor digitorum communis

figure 86

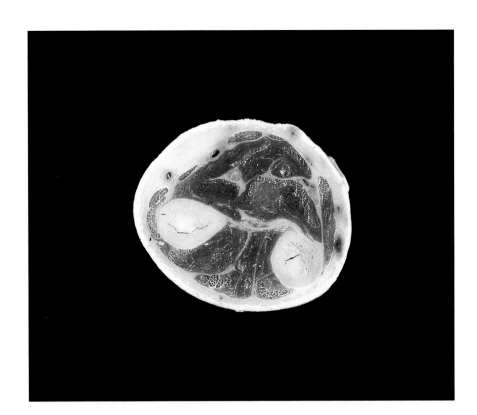

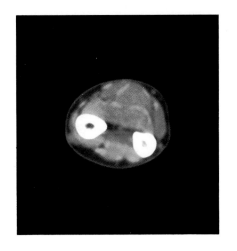

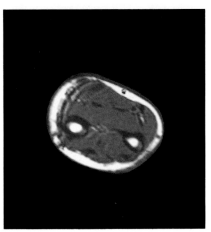

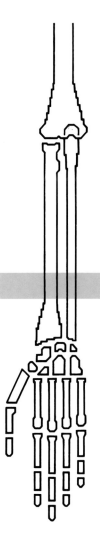

figure 87

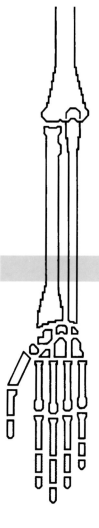

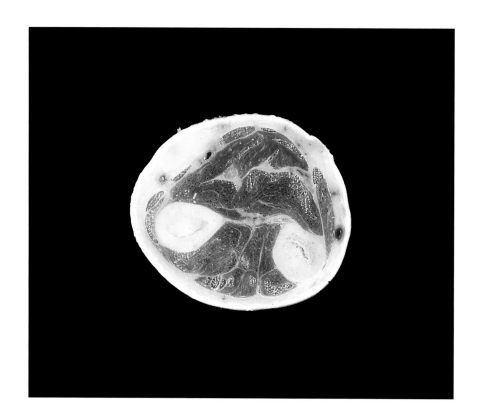

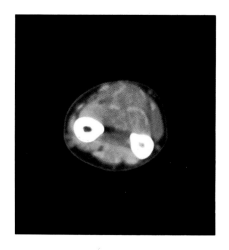

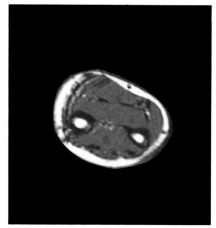

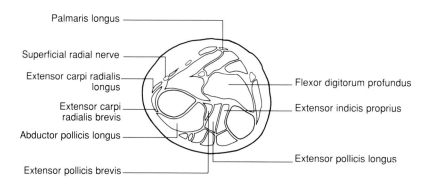

Palmaris longus

Superficial radial nerve

Extensor carpi radialis longus

Extensor carpi radialis brevis

Abductor pollicis longus

Extensor pollicis brevis

Flexor digitorum profundus

Extensor indicis proprius

Extensor pollicis longus

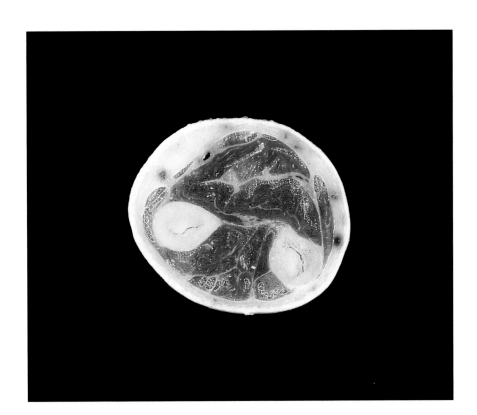

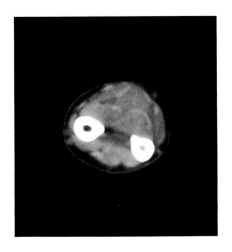

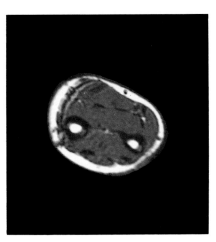

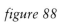
figure 88

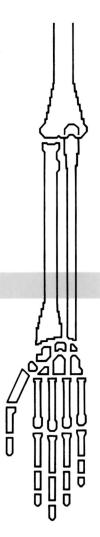

figure 89

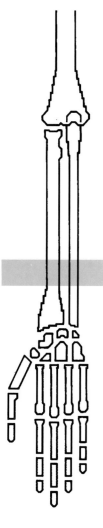

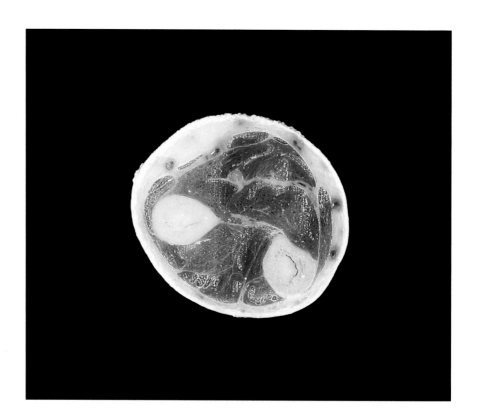

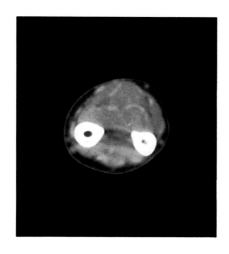

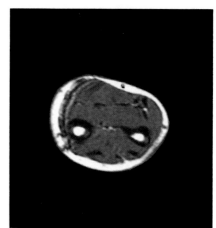

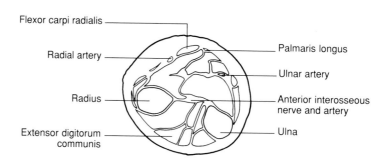

Flexor carpi radialis

Radial artery

Radius

Extensor digitorum communis

Palmaris longus

Ulnar artery

Anterior interosseous nerve and artery

Ulna

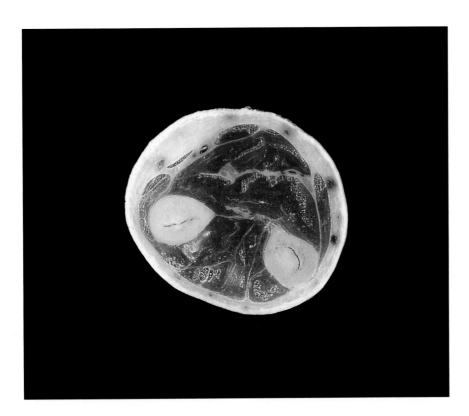

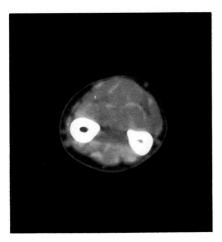

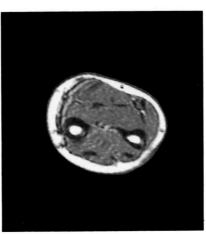

figure 90

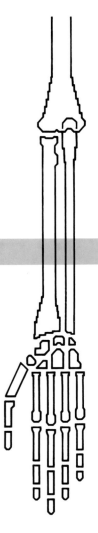

figure 91

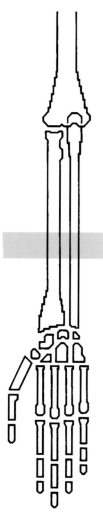

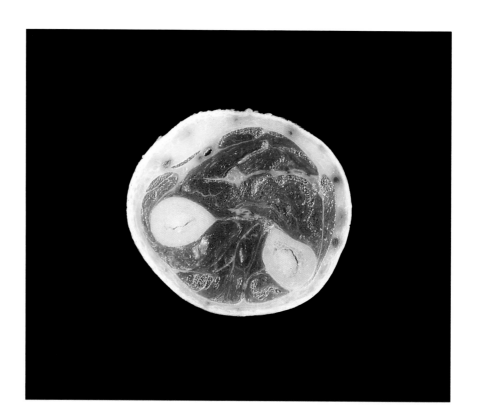

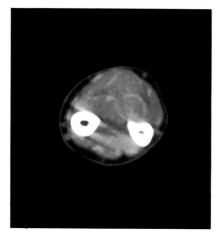

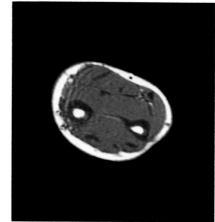

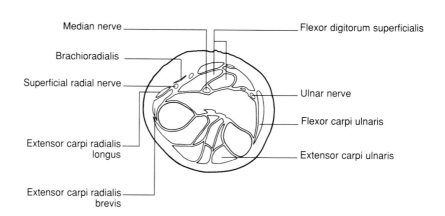

Median nerve — Flexor digitorum superficialis

Brachioradialis

Superficial radial nerve — Ulnar nerve

Flexor carpi ulnaris

Extensor carpi radialis longus — Extensor carpi ulnaris

Extensor carpi radialis brevis

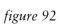

figure 92

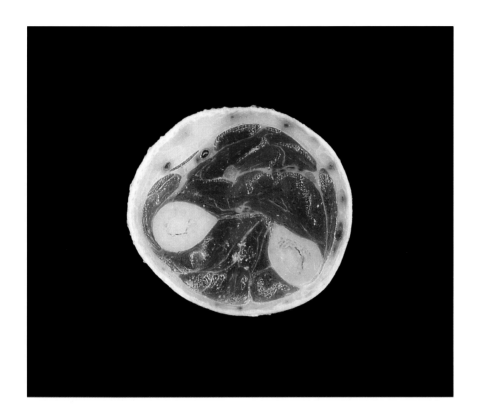

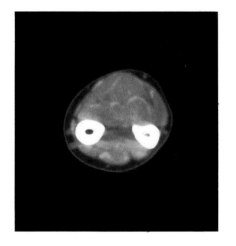

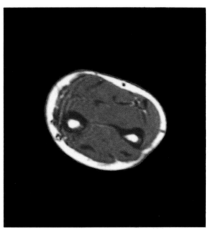

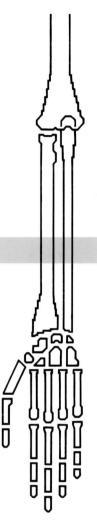

figure 93

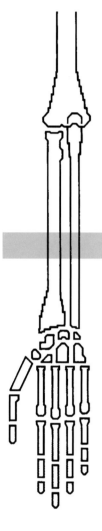

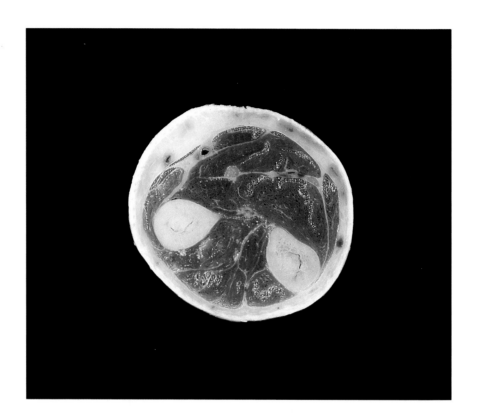

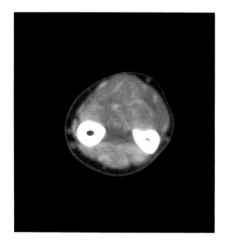

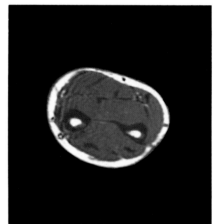

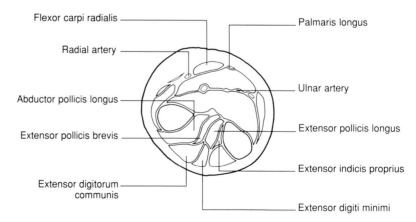

Flexor carpi radialis

Radial artery

Abductor pollicis longus

Extensor pollicis brevis

Extensor digitorum
communis

Palmaris longus

Ulnar artery

Extensor pollicis longus

Extensor indicis proprius

Extensor digiti minimi

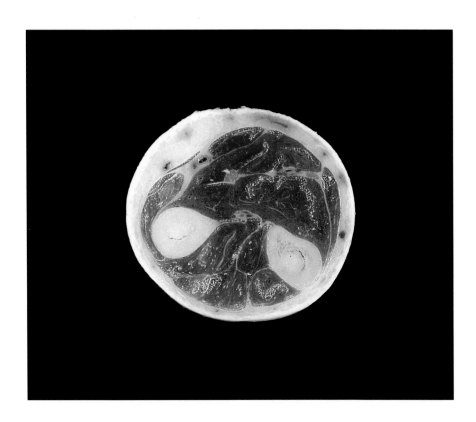

figure 94

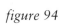

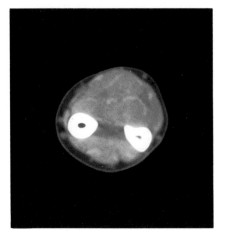

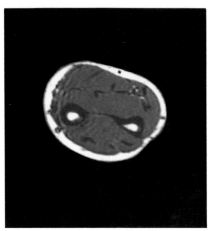

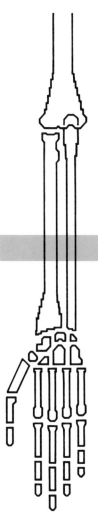

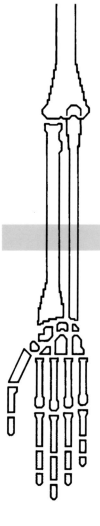

figure 95

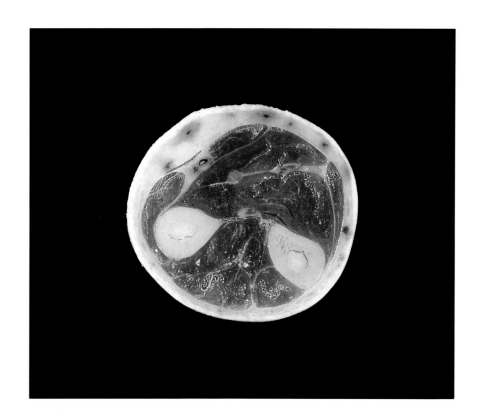

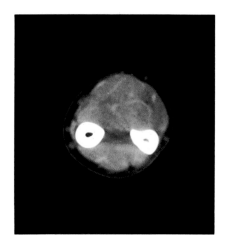

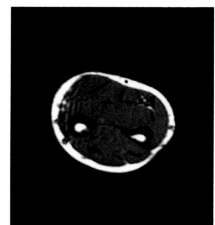

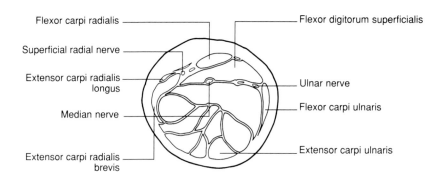

Flexor carpi radialis — | — Flexor digitorum superficialis

Superficial radial nerve —

Extensor carpi radialis longus —

Median nerve — | — Ulnar nerve

— Flexor carpi ulnaris

Extensor carpi radialis brevis —

— Extensor carpi ulnaris

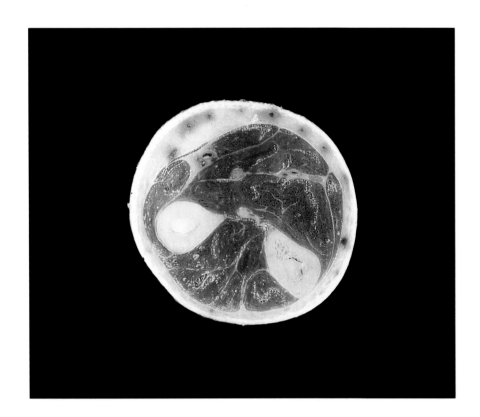

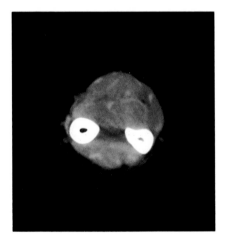

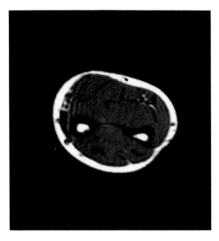

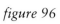

figure 96

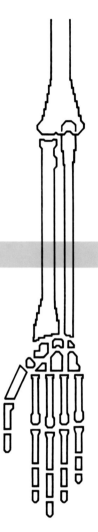

figure 97

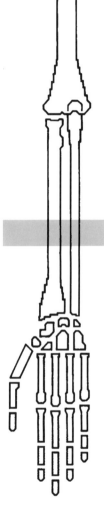

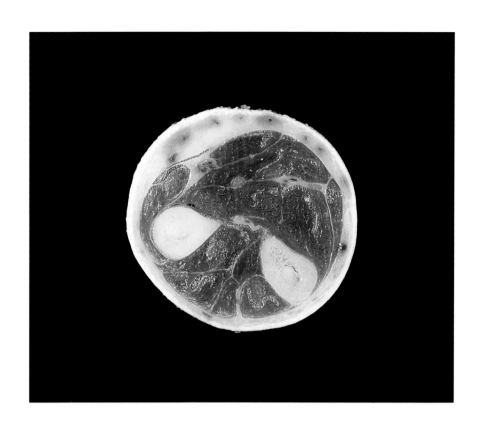

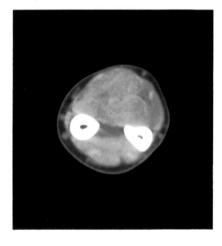

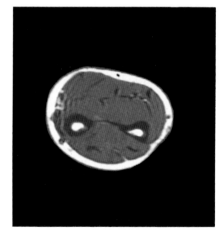

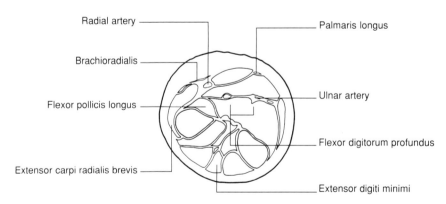

Radial artery

Brachioradialis

Flexor pollicis longus

Extensor carpi radialis brevis

Palmaris longus

Ulnar artery

Flexor digitorum profundus

Extensor digiti minimi

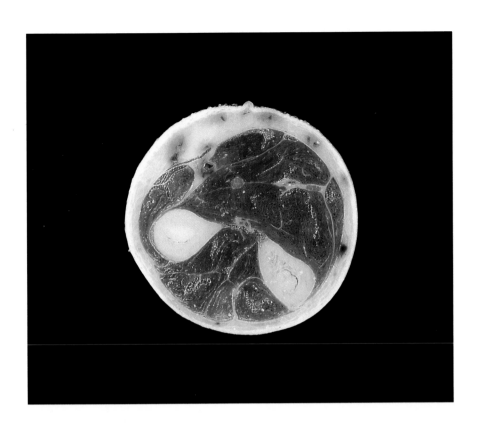

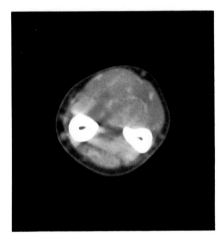

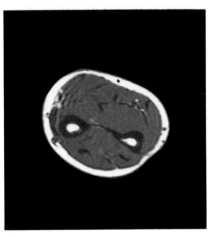

figure 98

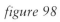

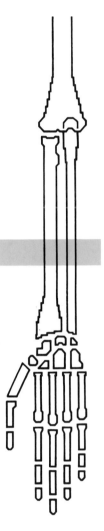

figure 99

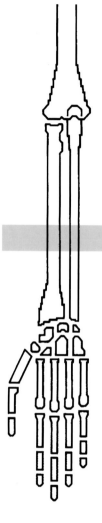

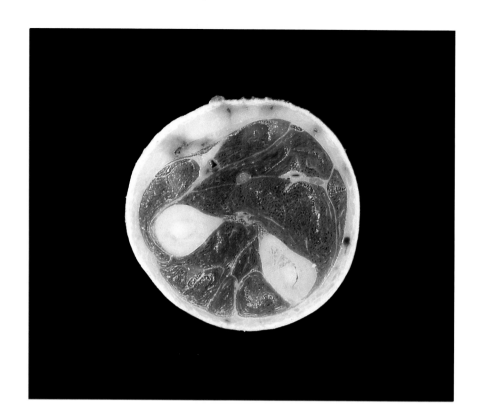

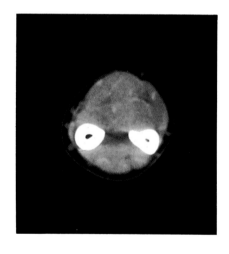

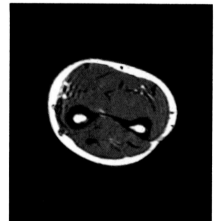

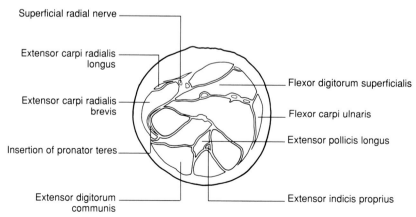

Superficial radial nerve

Extensor carpi radialis longus

Extensor carpi radialis brevis

Insertion of pronator teres

Extensor digitorum communis

Flexor digitorum superficialis

Flexor carpi ulnaris

Extensor pollicis longus

Extensor indicis proprius

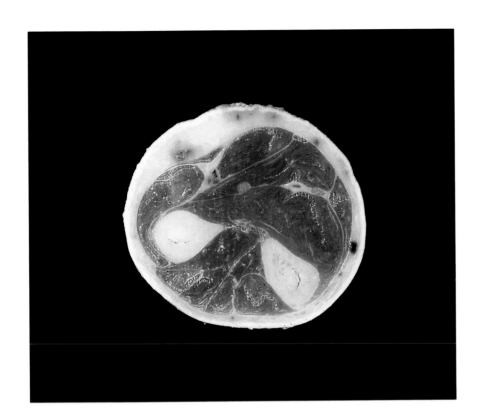

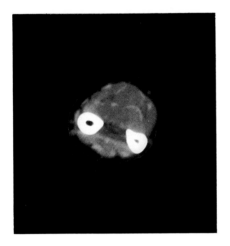

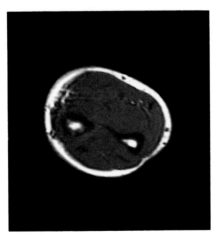

figure 100

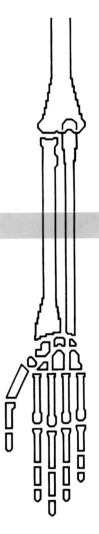

figure 101

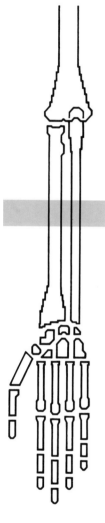

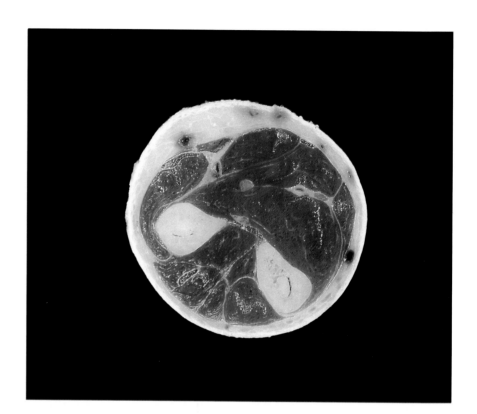

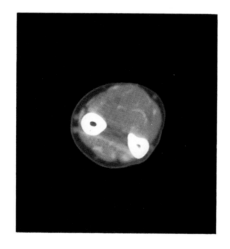

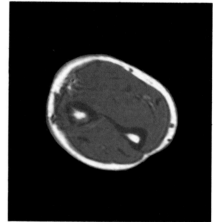

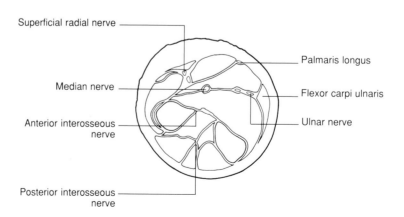

Superficial radial nerve

Median nerve

Anterior interosseous nerve

Posterior interosseous nerve

Palmaris longus

Flexor carpi ulnaris

Ulnar nerve

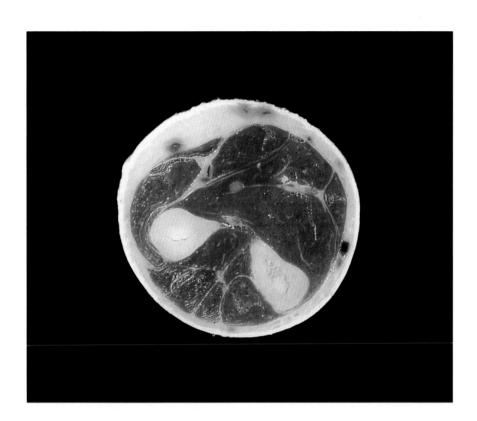

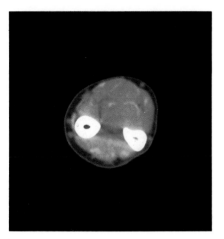

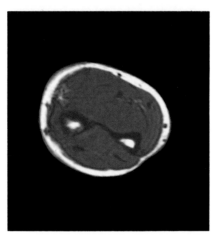

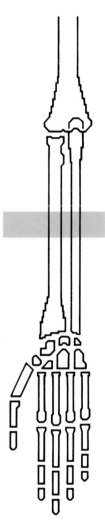

figure 102

figure 103

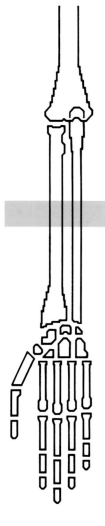

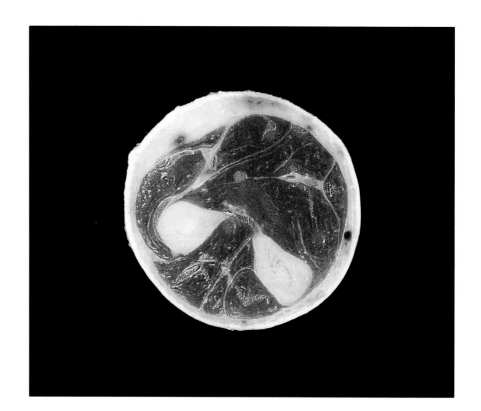

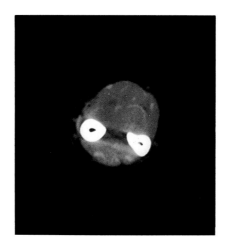

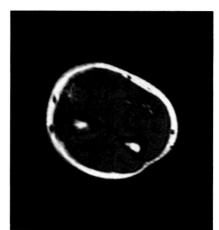

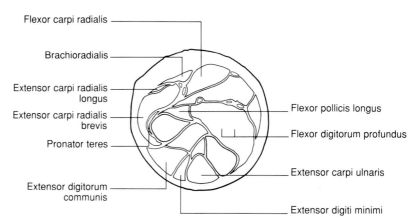

Flexor carpi radialis

Brachioradialis

Extensor carpi radialis
longus

Extensor carpi radialis
brevis

Pronator teres

Extensor digitorum
communis

Flexor pollicis longus

Flexor digitorum profundus

Extensor carpi ulnaris

Extensor digiti minimi

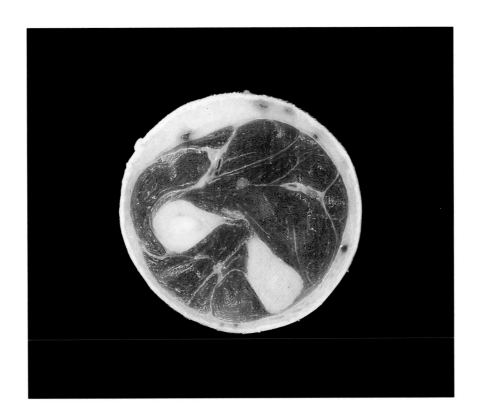

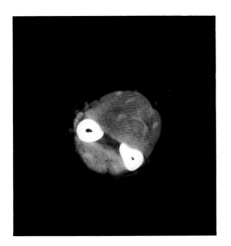

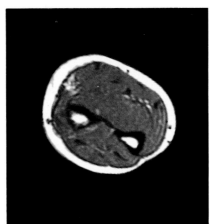

figure 104

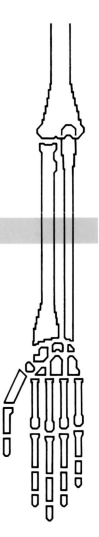

figure 105

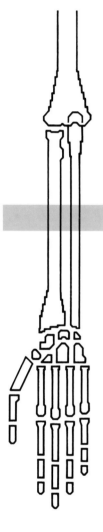

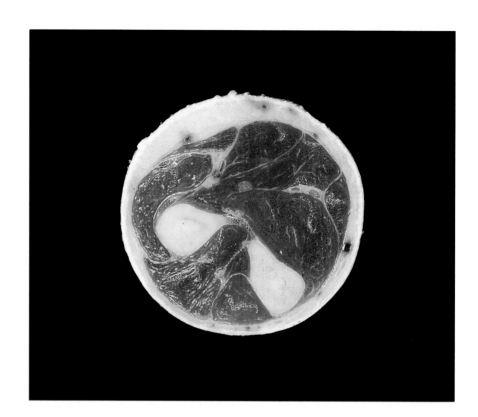

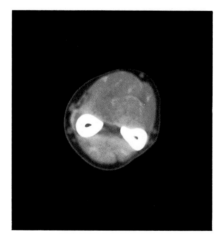

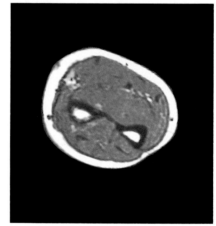

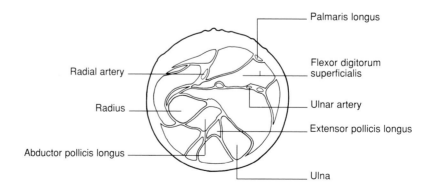

Palmaris longus

Flexor digitorum superficialis

Radial artery

Ulnar artery

Radius

Extensor pollicis longus

Abductor pollicis longus

Ulna

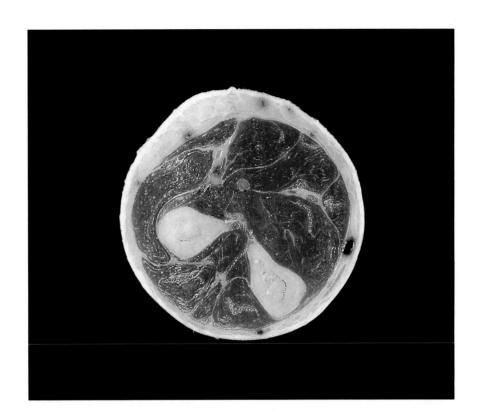

figure 106

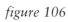

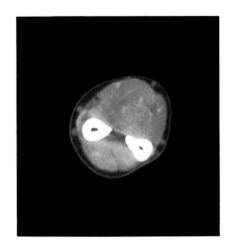

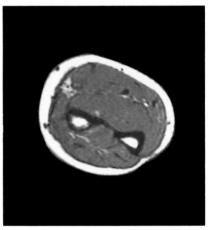

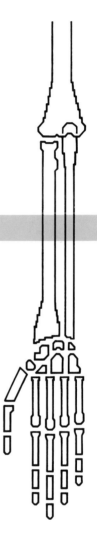

figure 107

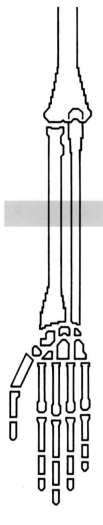

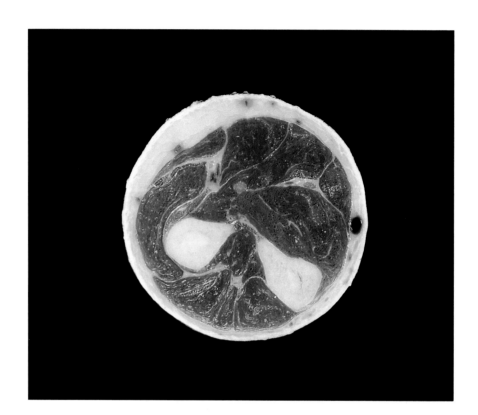

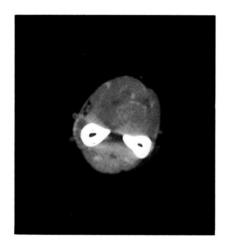

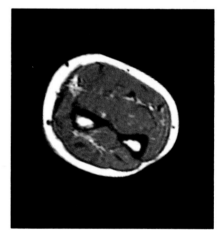

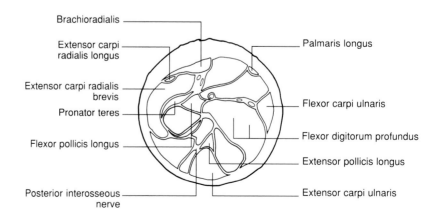

Brachioradialis

Extensor carpi radialis longus

Extensor carpi radialis brevis

Pronator teres

Flexor pollicis longus

Posterior interosseous nerve

Palmaris longus

Flexor carpi ulnaris

Flexor digitorum profundus

Extensor pollicis longus

Extensor carpi ulnaris

figure 108

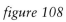

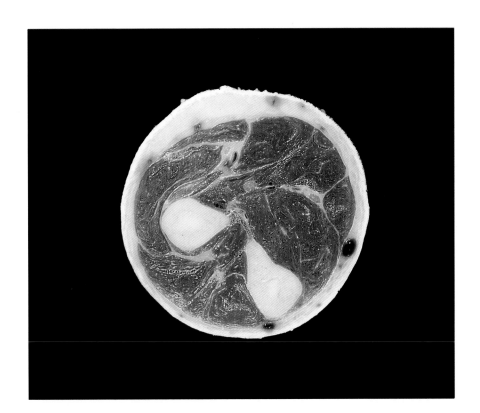

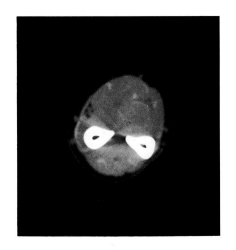

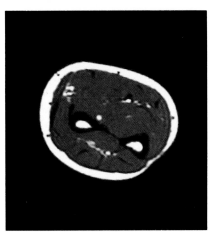

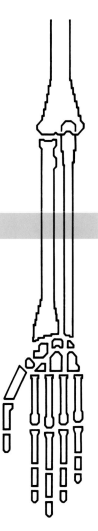

figure 109

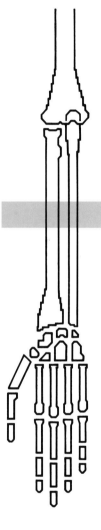

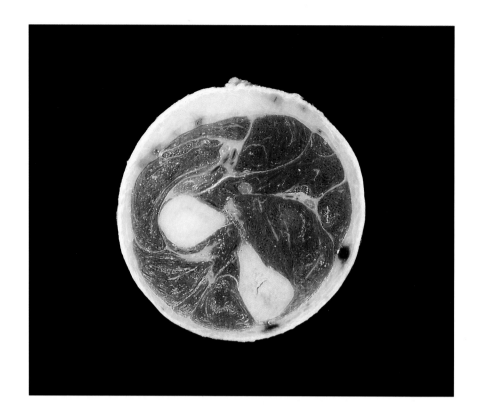

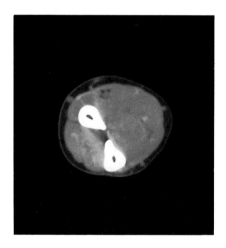

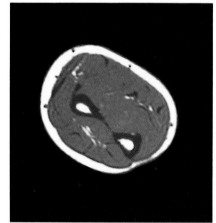

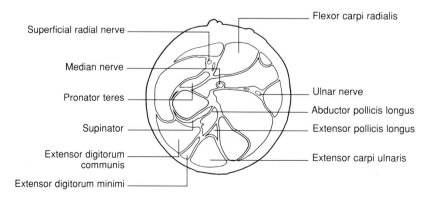

Superficial radial nerve

Median nerve

Pronator teres

Supinator

Extensor digitorum communis

Extensor digitorum minimi

Flexor carpi radialis

Ulnar nerve

Abductor pollicis longus

Extensor pollicis longus

Extensor carpi ulnaris

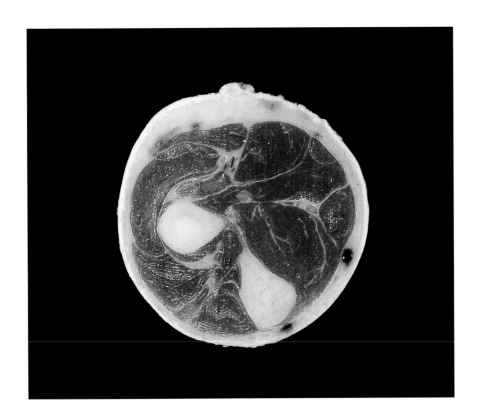

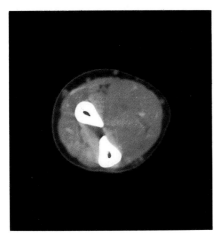 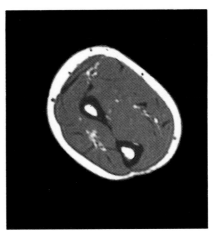

figure 110

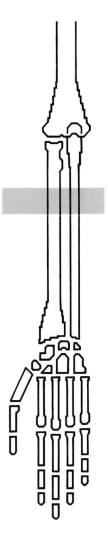

figure 111

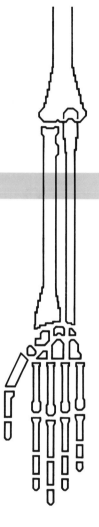

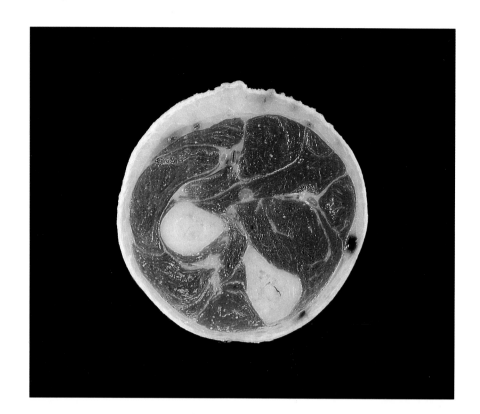

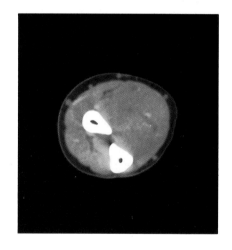

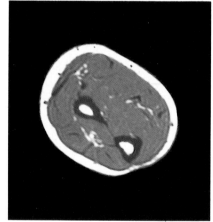

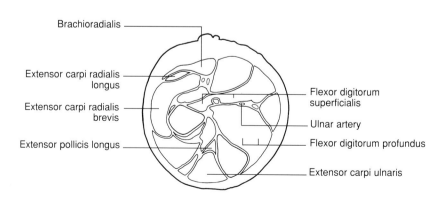

Brachioradialis

Extensor carpi radialis
longus

Extensor carpi radialis
brevis

Extensor pollicis longus

Flexor digitorum
superficialis

Ulnar artery

Flexor digitorum profundus

Extensor carpi ulnaris

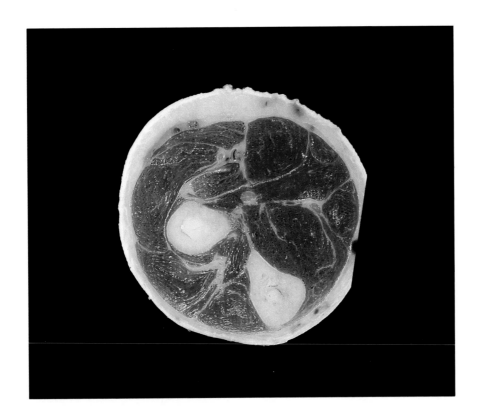

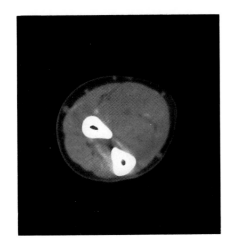

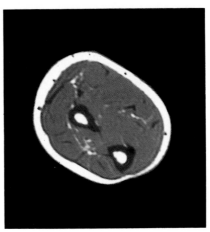

figure 112

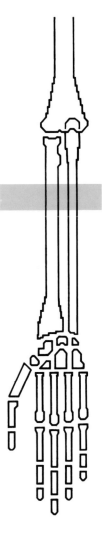

figure 113

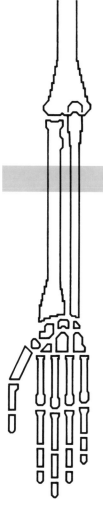

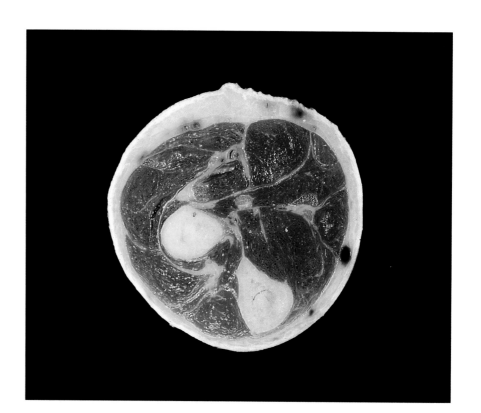

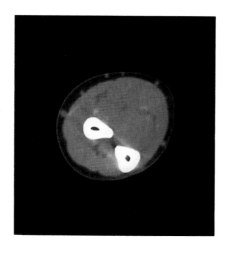

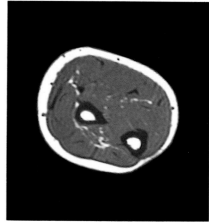

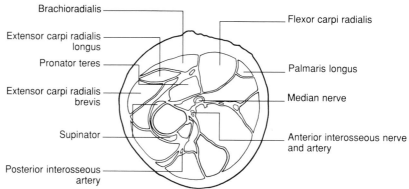

Brachioradialis

Extensor carpi radialis longus

Pronator teres

Extensor carpi radialis brevis

Supinator

Posterior interosseous artery

Flexor carpi radialis

Palmaris longus

Median nerve

Anterior interosseous nerve and artery

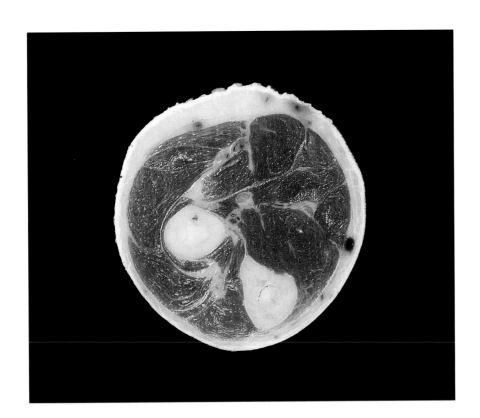

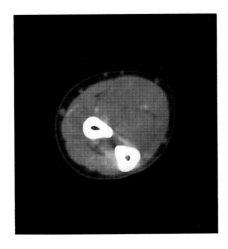

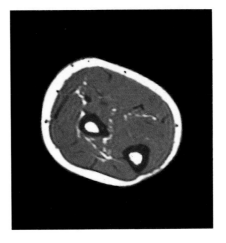

figure 114

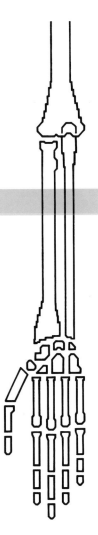

figure 115

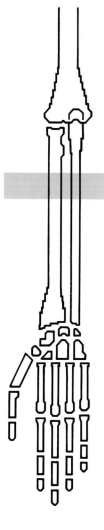

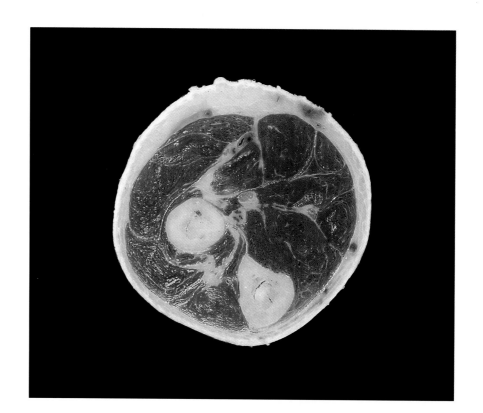

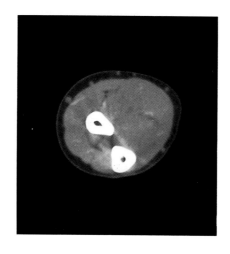
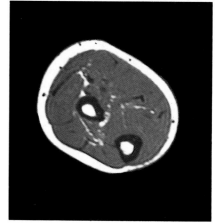

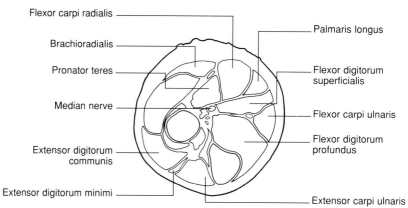

Flexor carpi radialis

Brachioradialis

Pronator teres

Median nerve

Extensor digitorum communis

Extensor digitorum minimi

Palmaris longus

Flexor digitorum superficialis

Flexor carpi ulnaris

Flexor digitorum profundus

Extensor carpi ulnaris

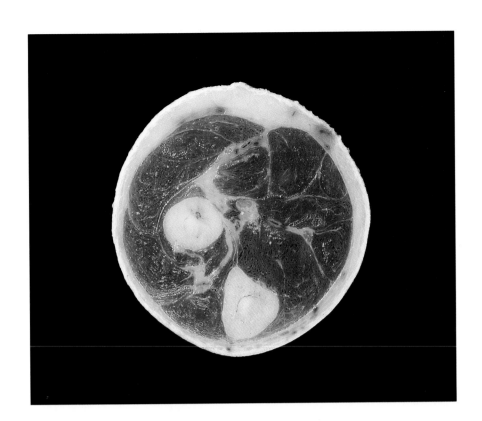

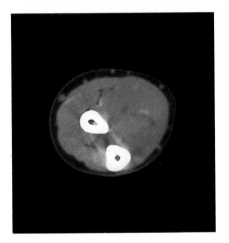

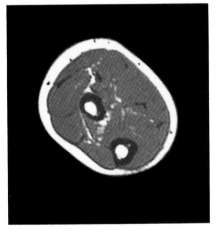

figure 116

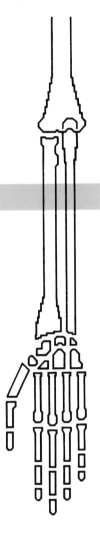

figure 117

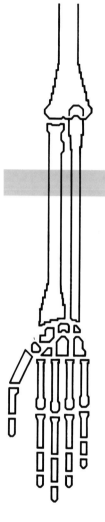

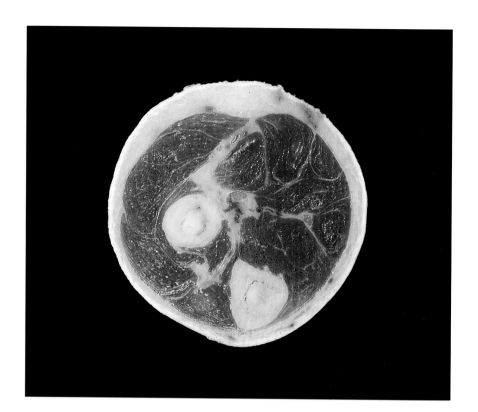

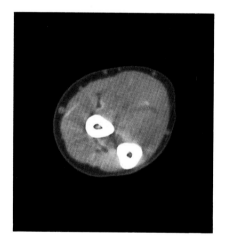

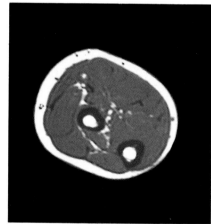

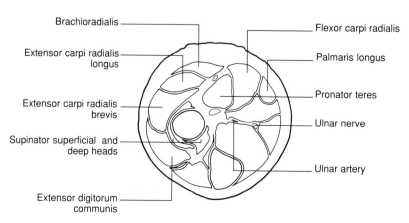

Brachioradialis

Extensor carpi radialis
longus

Extensor carpi radialis
brevis

Supinator superficial and
deep heads

Extensor digitorum
communis

Flexor carpi radialis

Palmaris longus

Pronator teres

Ulnar nerve

Ulnar artery

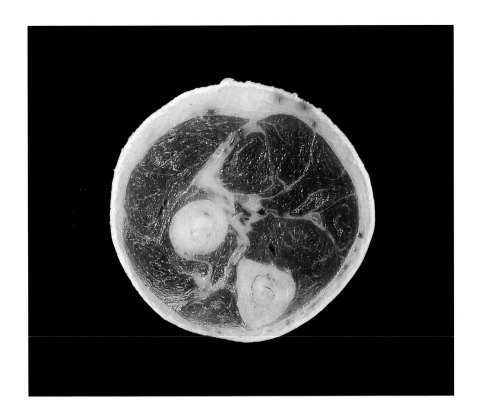

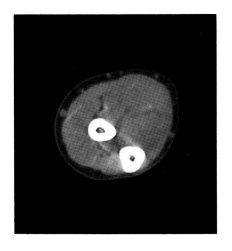

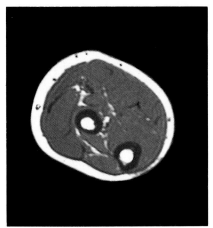

figure 118

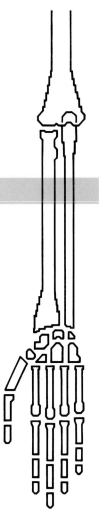

figure 119

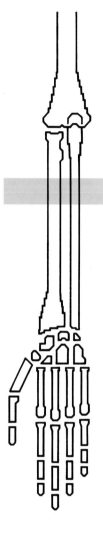

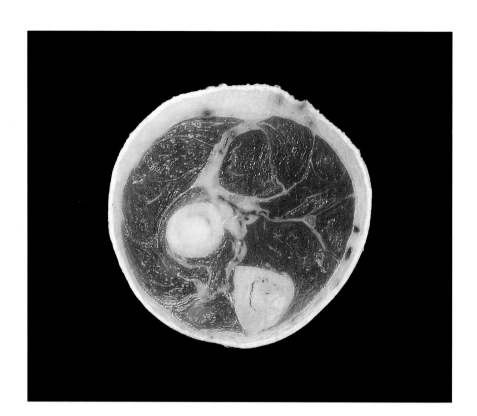

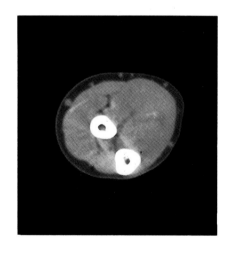

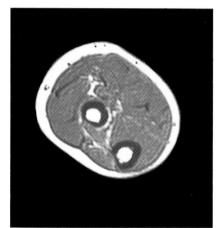

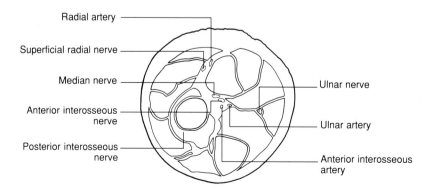

Radial artery

Superficial radial nerve

Median nerve

Anterior interosseous
nerve

Posterior interosseous
nerve

Ulnar nerve

Ulnar artery

Anterior interosseous
artery

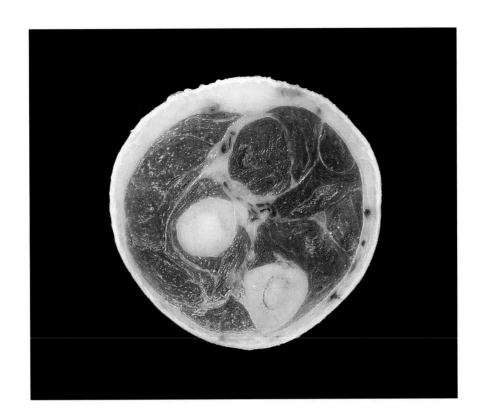

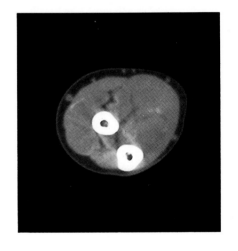

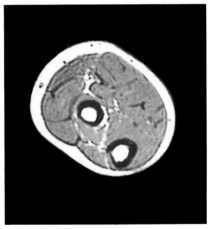

figure 120

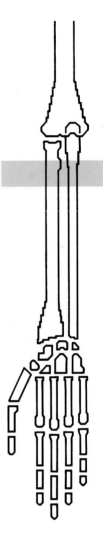

figure 121

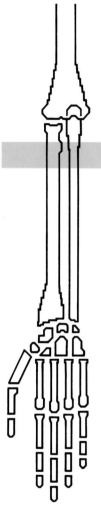

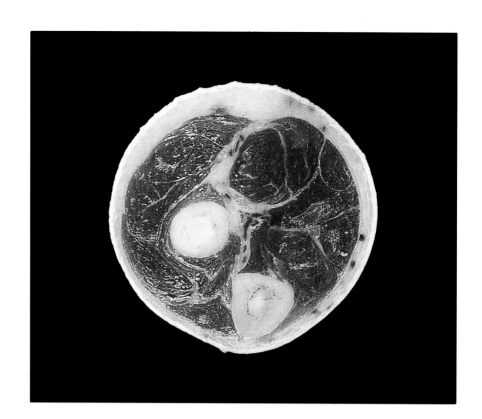

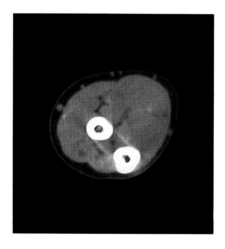

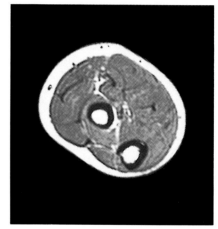

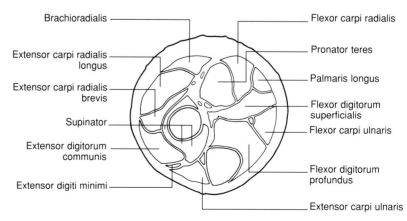

Brachioradialis — Flexor carpi radialis

Extensor carpi radialis longus — Pronator teres

Extensor carpi radialis brevis — Palmaris longus

Supinator — Flexor digitorum superficialis

Flexor carpi ulnaris

Extensor digitorum communis

Flexor digitorum profundus

Extensor digiti minimi

Extensor carpi ulnaris

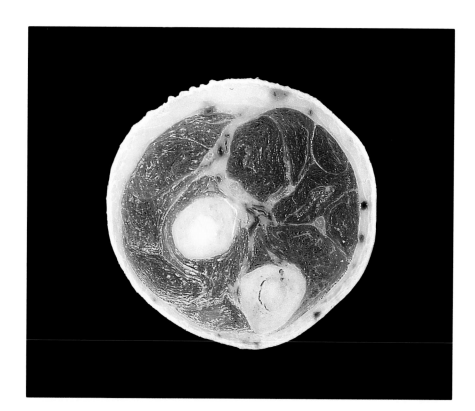

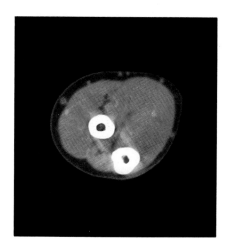

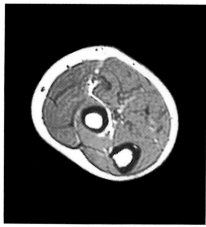

figure 122

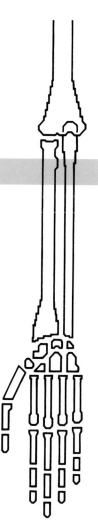

figure 123

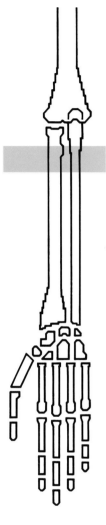

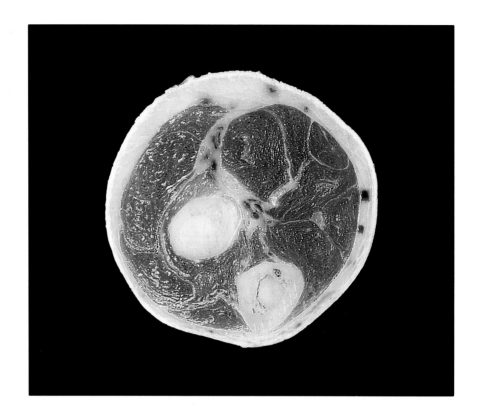

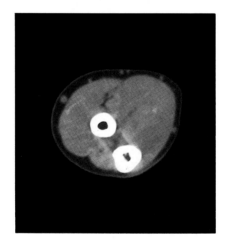

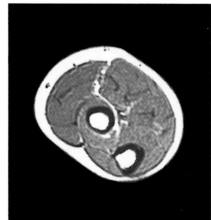

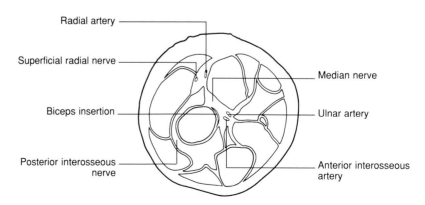

Radial artery

Superficial radial nerve

Median nerve

Biceps insertion

Ulnar artery

Posterior interosseous nerve

Anterior interosseous artery

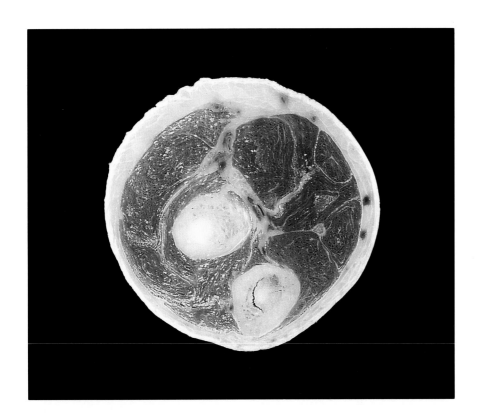

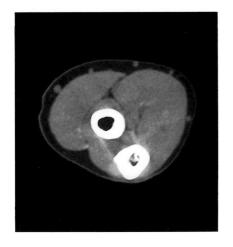

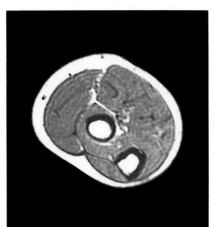

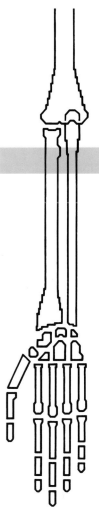

figure 124

figure 125

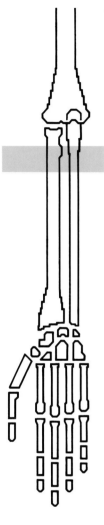

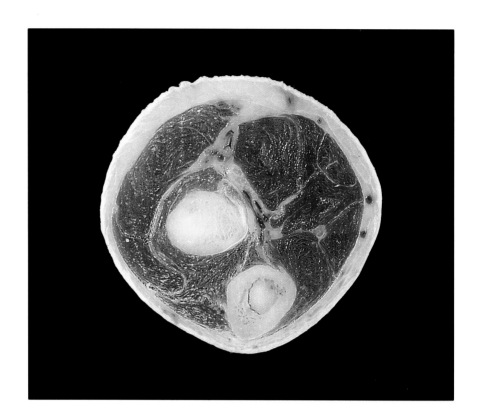

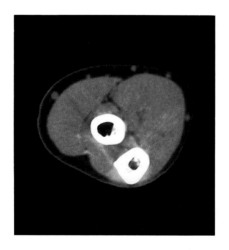

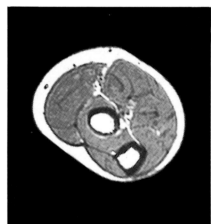

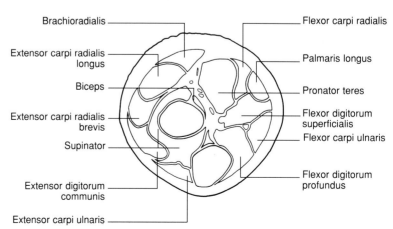

Brachioradialis

Extensor carpi radialis longus

Biceps

Extensor carpi radialis brevis

Supinator

Extensor digitorum communis

Extensor carpi ulnaris

Flexor carpi radialis

Palmaris longus

Pronator teres

Flexor digitorum superficialis

Flexor carpi ulnaris

Flexor digitorum profundus

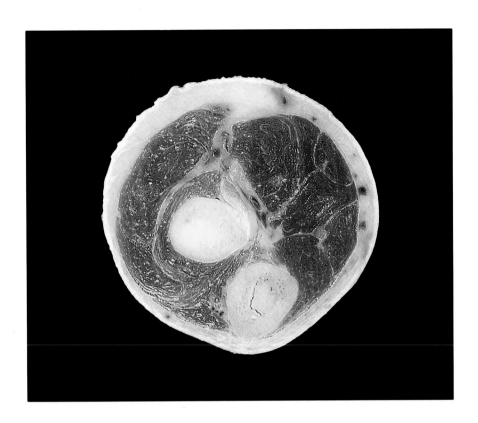

figure 126

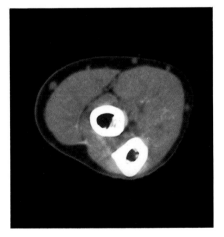

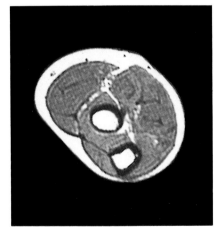

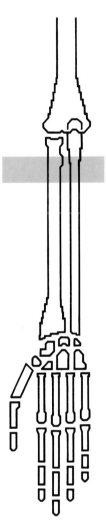

figure 127

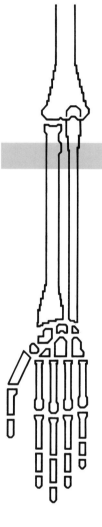

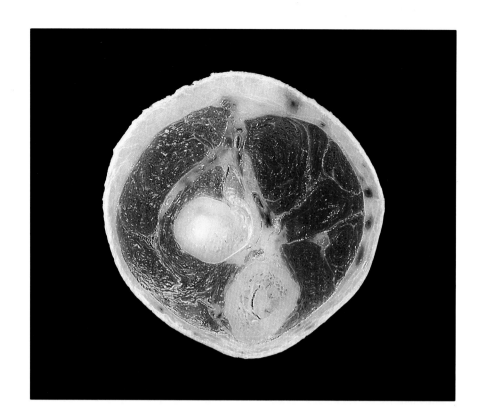

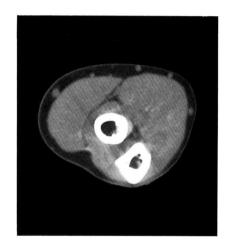

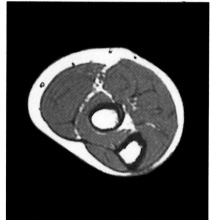

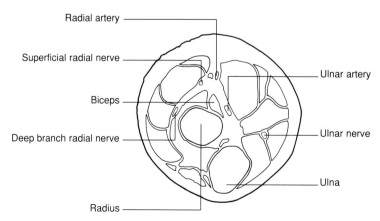

Radial artery

Superficial radial nerve

Biceps

Deep branch radial nerve

Radius

Ulnar artery

Ulnar nerve

Ulna

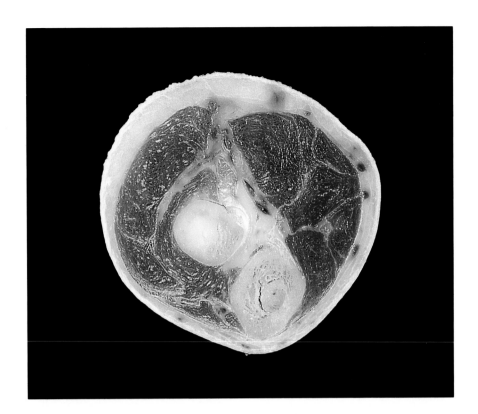

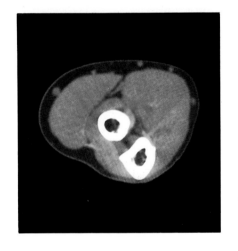

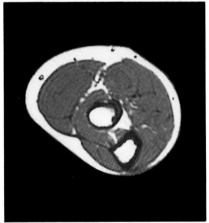

figure 128

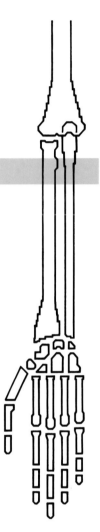

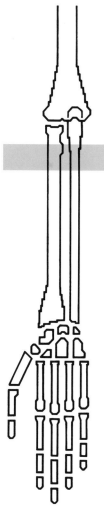

figure 129

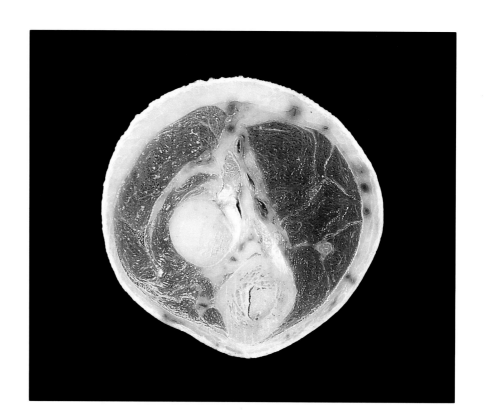

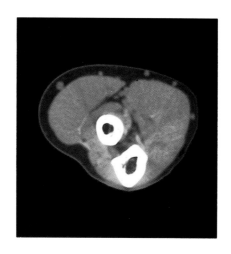

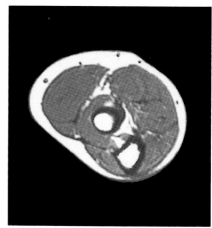

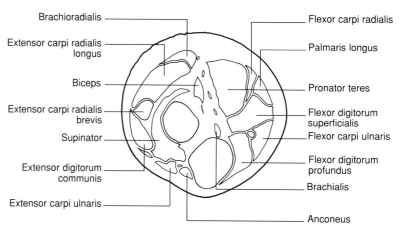

Brachioradialis

Extensor carpi radialis longus

Biceps

Extensor carpi radialis brevis

Supinator

Extensor digitorum communis

Extensor carpi ulnaris

Flexor carpi radialis

Palmaris longus

Pronator teres

Flexor digitorum superficialis

Flexor carpi ulnaris

Flexor digitorum profundus

Brachialis

Anconeus

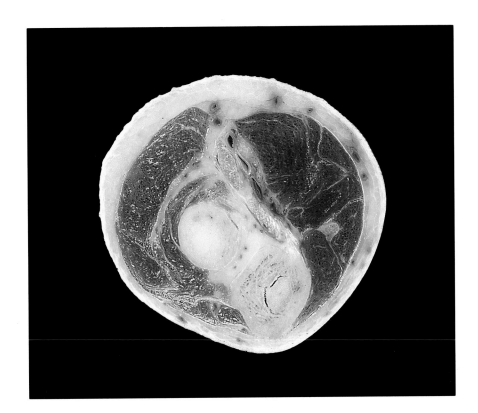

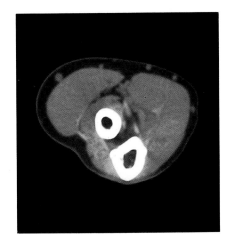

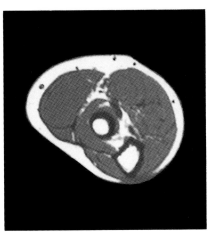

figure 130

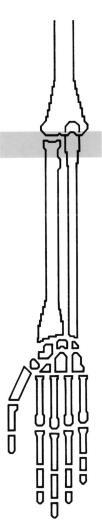

figure 131

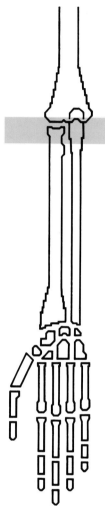

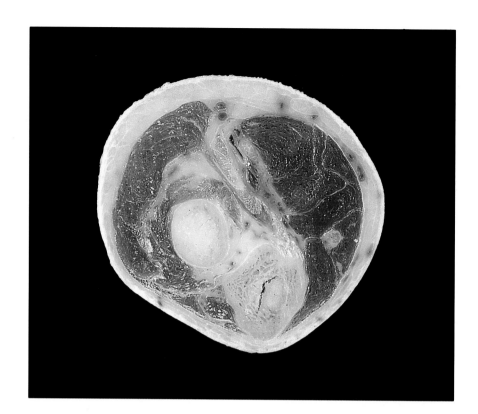

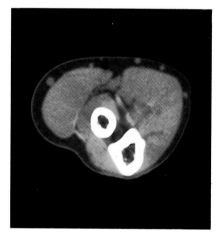

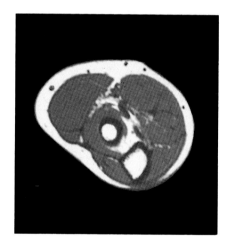

Lateral antebrachial cutaneous nerve

Biceps

Deep and superficial branches of radial nerve

Extensor digitorum communis

Extensor carpi ulnaris

Median nerve

Brachial artery

Brachialis

Ulnar nerve

Anconeus

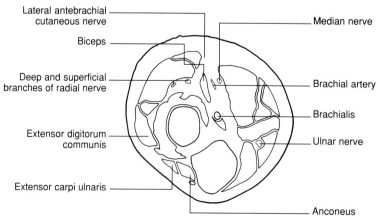

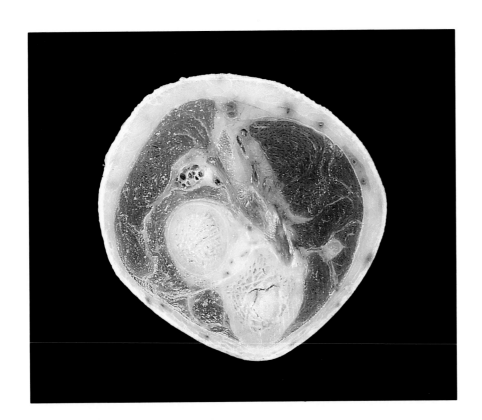

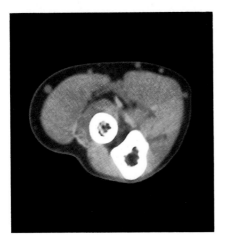

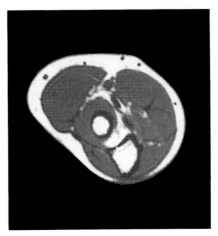

figure 132

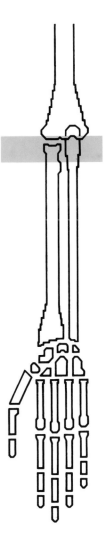

figure 133

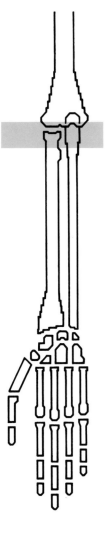

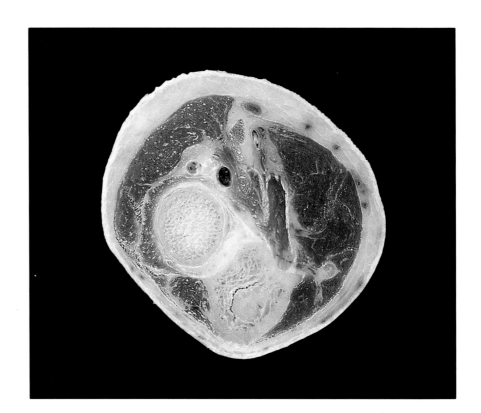

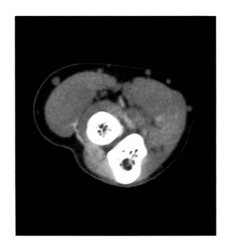

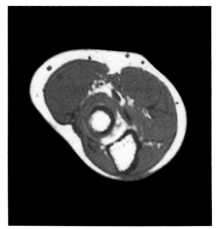

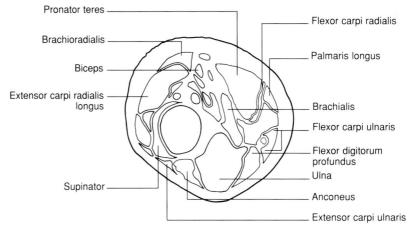

Pronator teres

Brachioradialis

Biceps

Extensor carpi radialis
longus

Supinator

Flexor carpi radialis

Palmaris longus

Brachialis

Flexor carpi ulnaris

Flexor digitorum
profundus

Ulna

Anconeus

Extensor carpi ulnaris

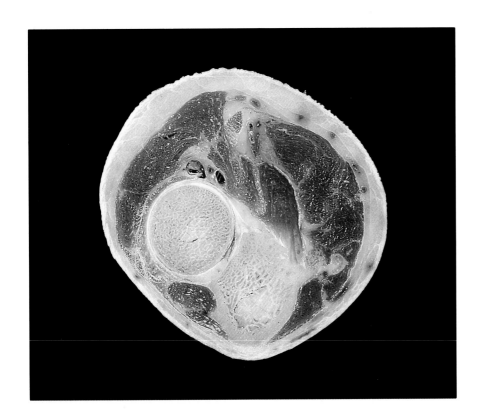

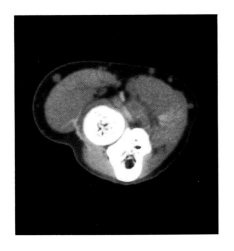
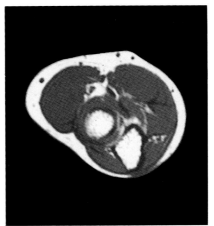

figure 134

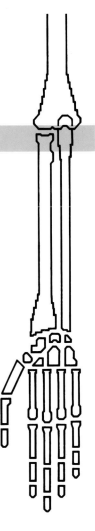

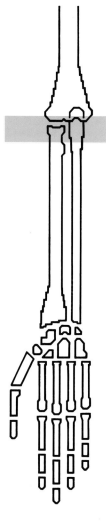

figure 135

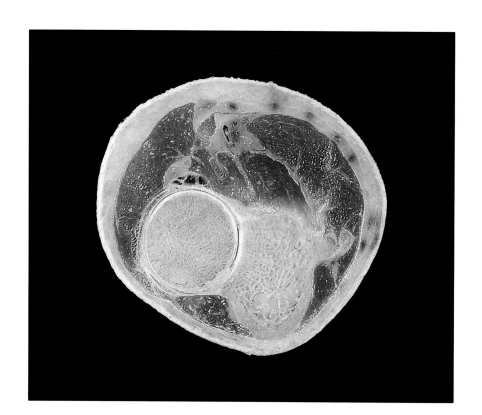

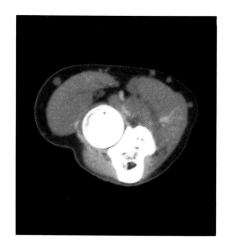

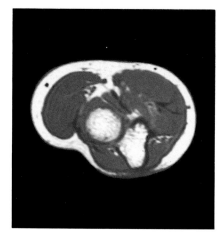

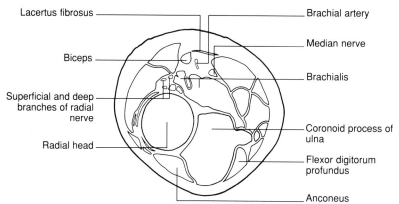

Lacertus fibrosus

Biceps

Superficial and deep branches of radial nerve

Radial head

Brachial artery

Median nerve

Brachialis

Coronoid process of ulna

Flexor digitorum profundus

Anconeus

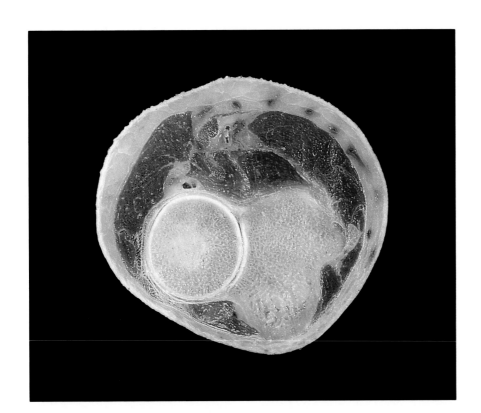

figure 136

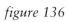

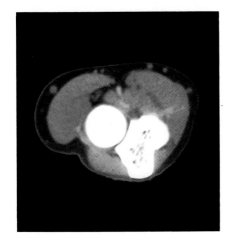

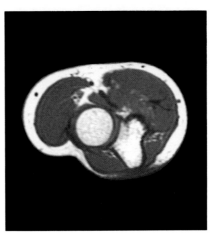

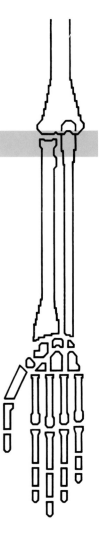

figure 137

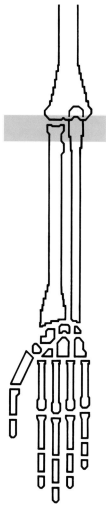

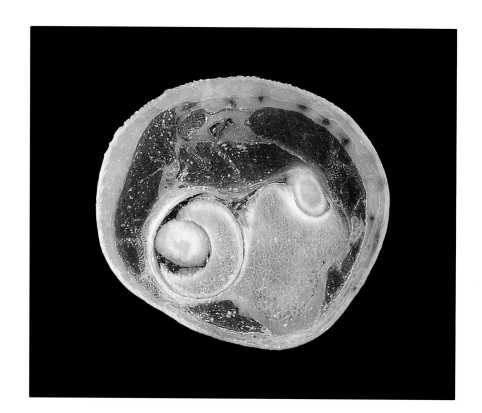

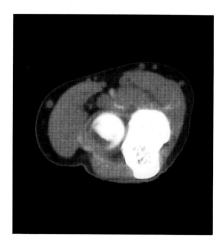

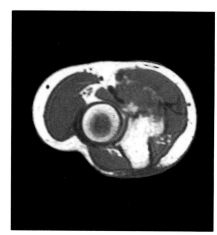

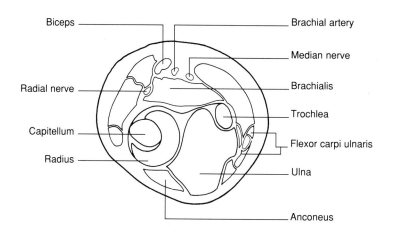

Biceps

Brachial artery

Median nerve

Radial nerve

Brachialis

Trochlea

Capitellum

Flexor carpi ulnaris

Radius

Ulna

Anconeus

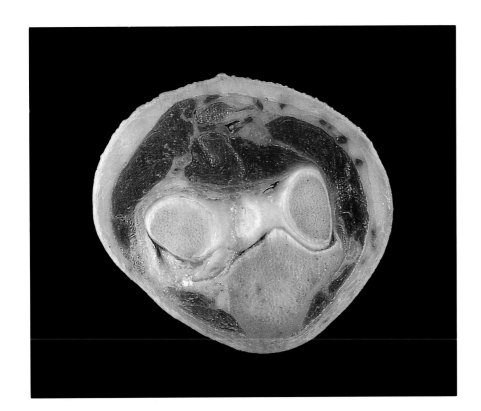

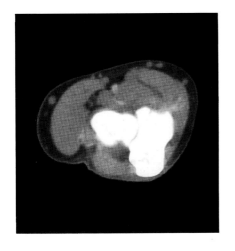

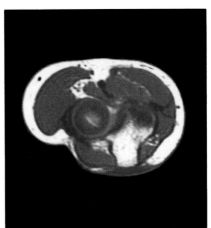

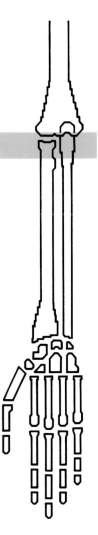

figure 138

figure 139

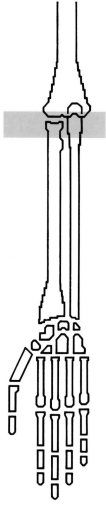

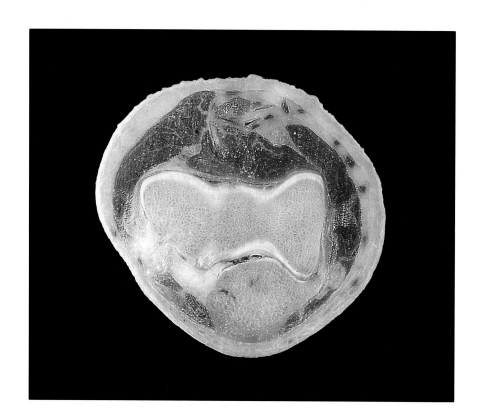

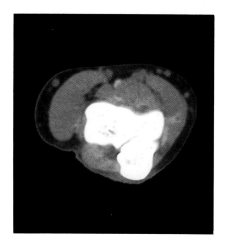

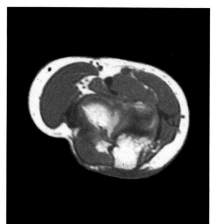

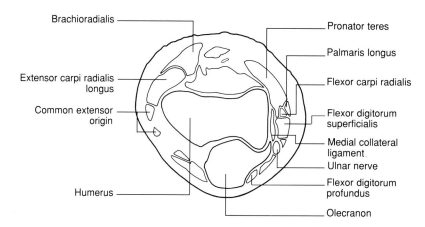

Brachioradialis

Extensor carpi radialis longus

Common extensor origin

Humerus

Pronator teres

Palmaris longus

Flexor carpi radialis

Flexor digitorum superficialis

Medial collateral ligament

Ulnar nerve

Flexor digitorum profundus

Olecranon

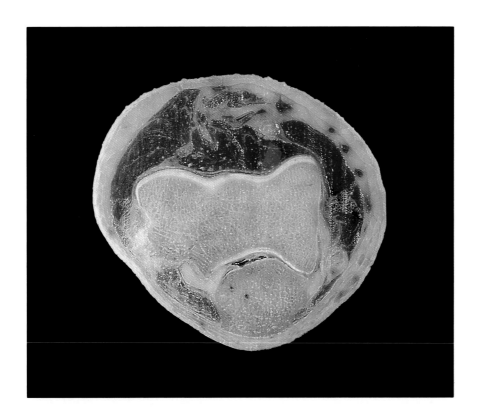

figure 140

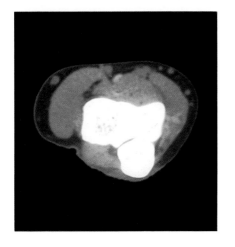

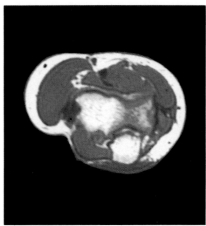

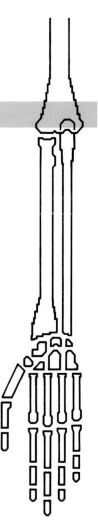

figure 141

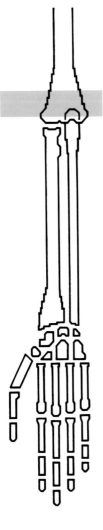

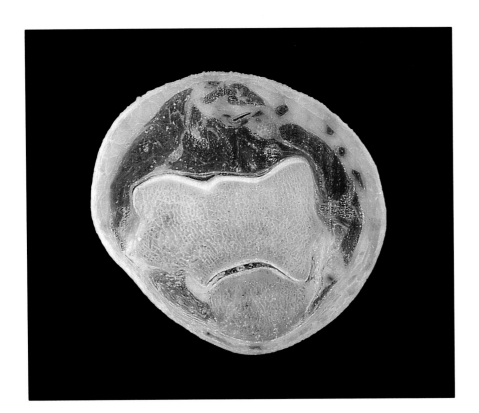

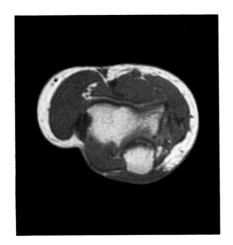

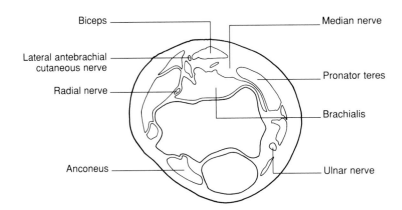

Biceps

Median nerve

Lateral antebrachial
cutaneous nerve

Radial nerve

Pronator teres

Brachialis

Anconeus

Ulnar nerve

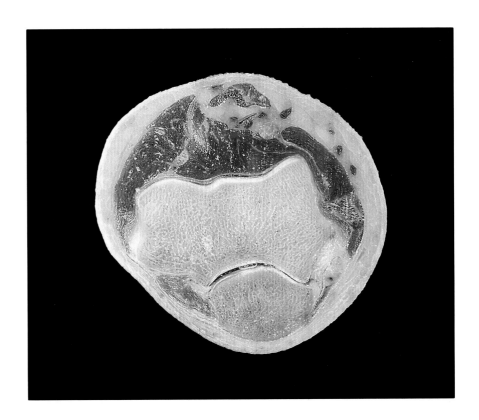

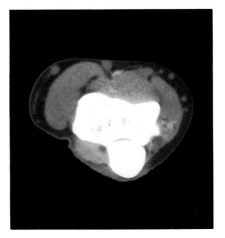

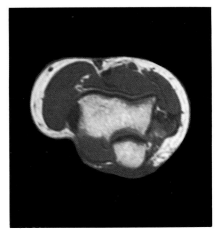

figure 142

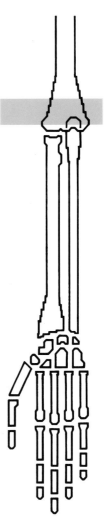

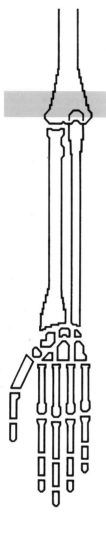

figure 143

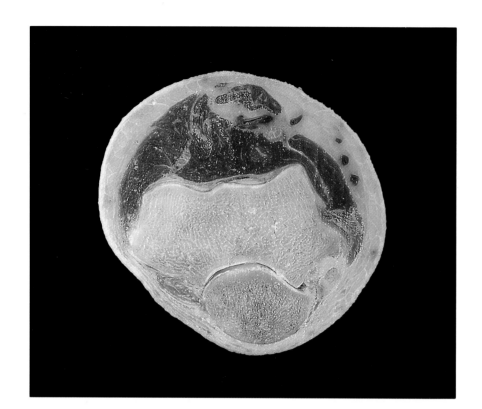

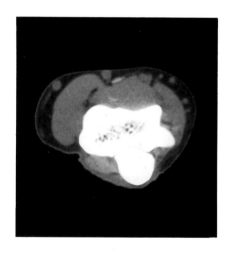

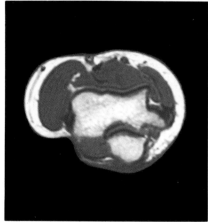

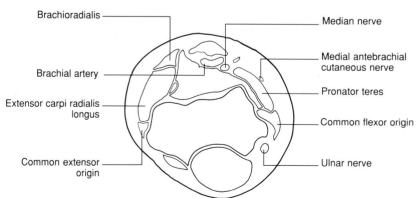

Brachioradialis

Median nerve

Brachial artery

Medial antebrachial
cutaneous nerve

Extensor carpi radialis
longus

Pronator teres

Common flexor origin

Common extensor
origin

Ulnar nerve

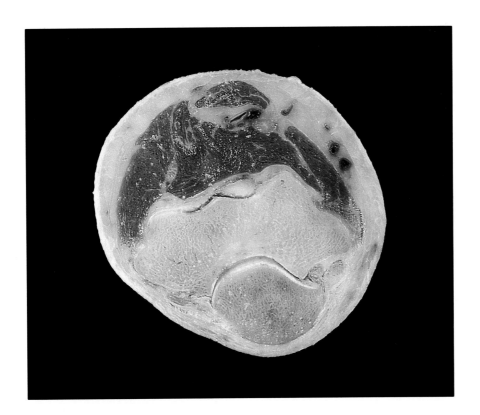

figure 144

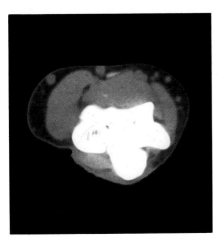

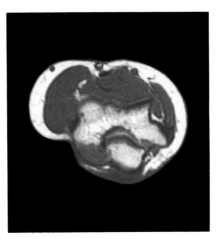

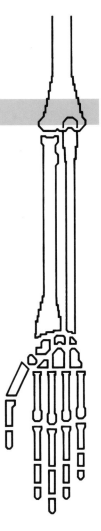

figure 145

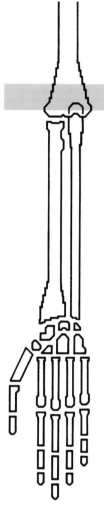

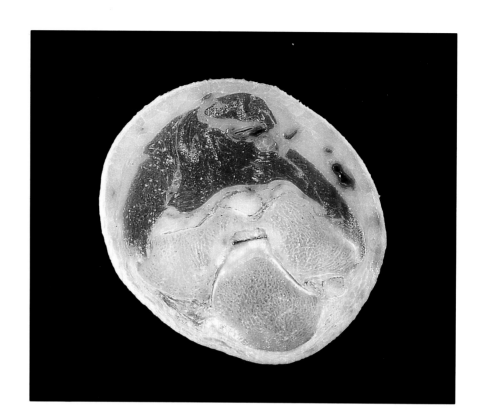

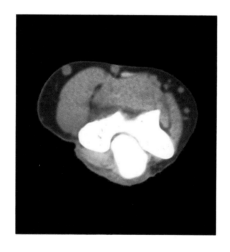

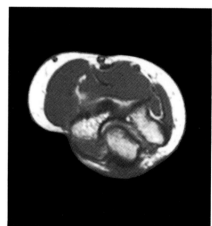

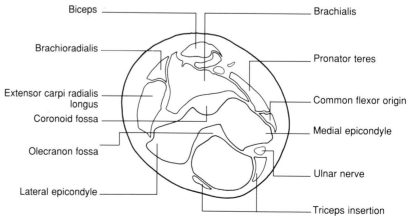

Biceps — Brachialis

Brachioradialis — Pronator teres

Extensor carpi radialis longus — Common flexor origin

Coronoid fossa — Medial epicondyle

Olecranon fossa — Ulnar nerve

Lateral epicondyle — Triceps insertion

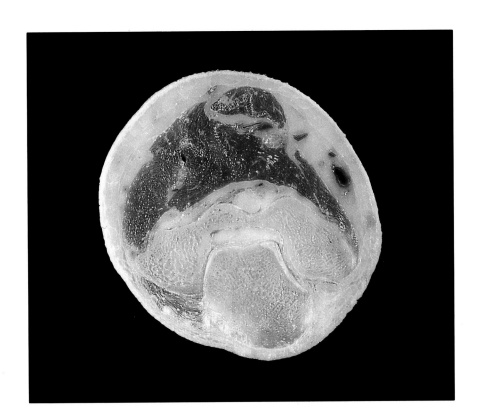

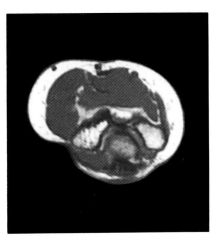

figure 146

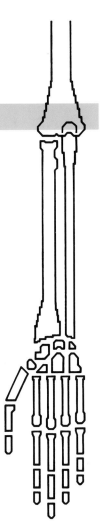

figure 147

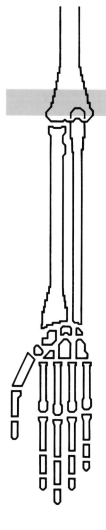

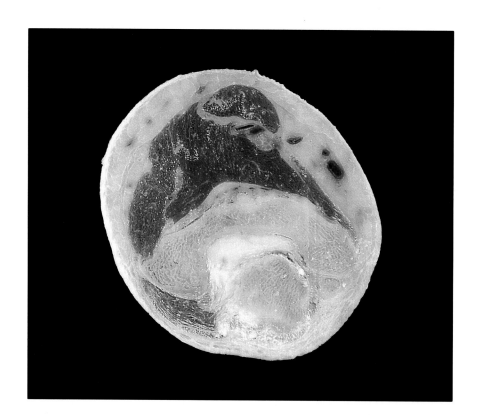

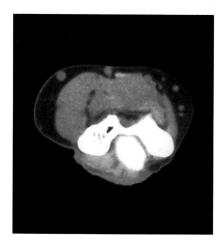

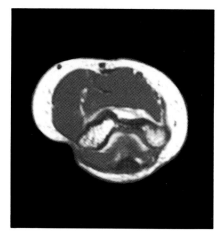

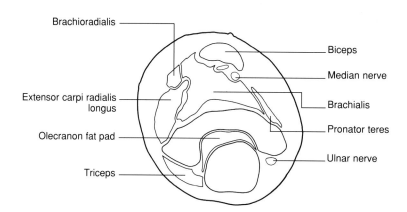

Brachioradialis

Extensor carpi radialis
longus

Olecranon fat pad

Triceps

Biceps

Median nerve

Brachialis

Pronator teres

Ulnar nerve

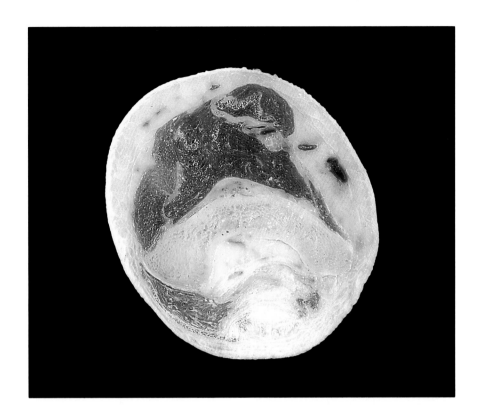

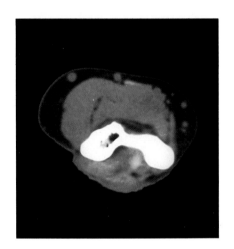
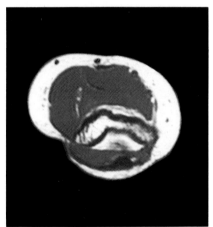

figure 148

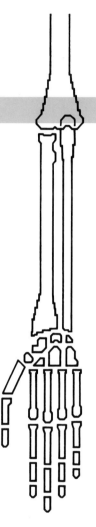

figure 149

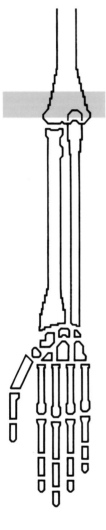

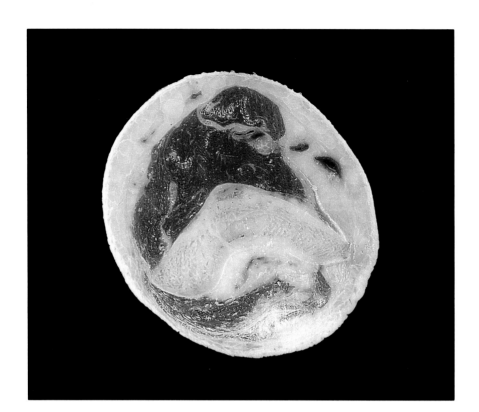

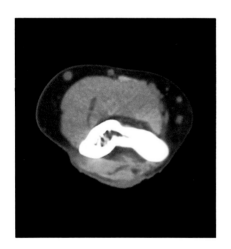

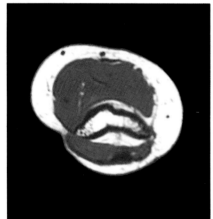

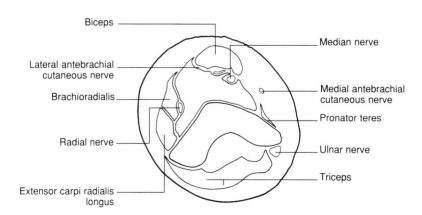

Biceps

Median nerve

Lateral antebrachial
cutaneous nerve

Brachioradialis

Medial antebrachial
cutaneous nerve

Pronator teres

Radial nerve

Ulnar nerve

Triceps

Extensor carpi radialis
longus

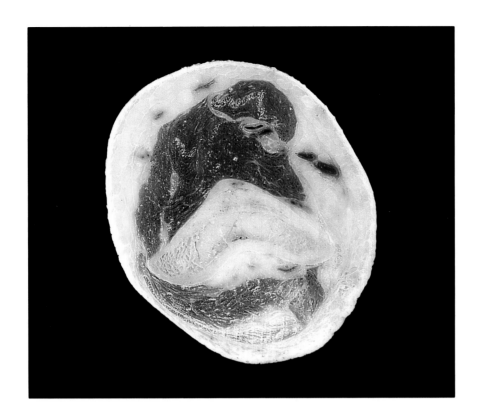

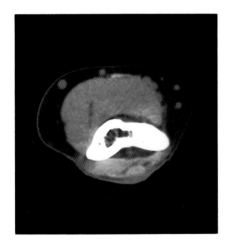 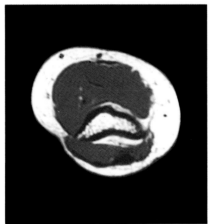

figure 150

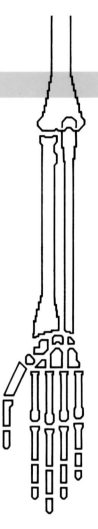

figure 151

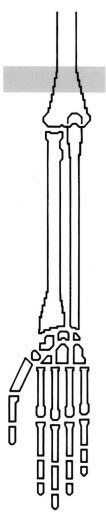

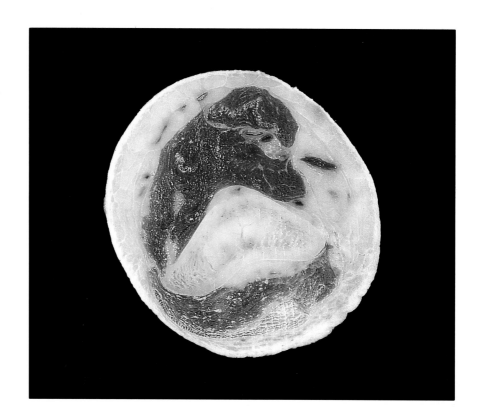

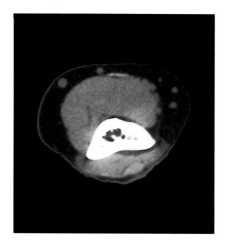

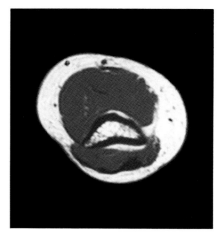

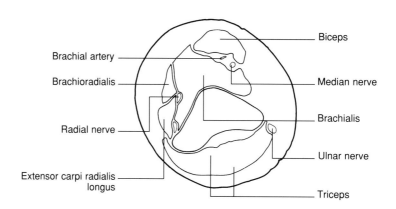

Brachial artery

Brachioradialis

Radial nerve

Extensor carpi radialis
longus

Biceps

Median nerve

Brachialis

Ulnar nerve

Triceps

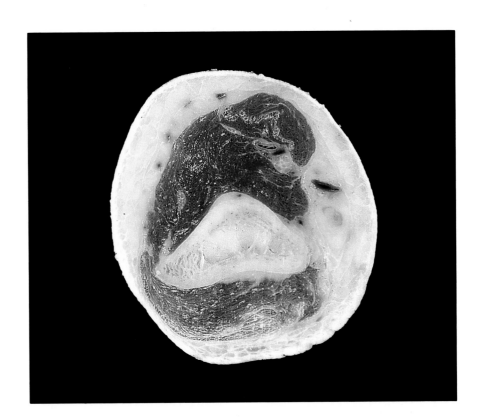

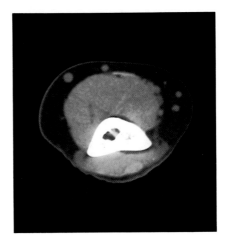
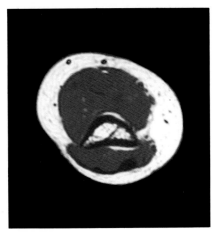

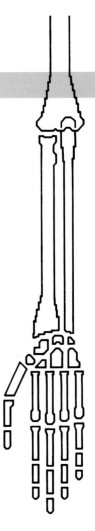

figure 152

figure 153

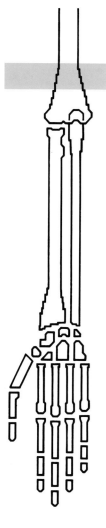

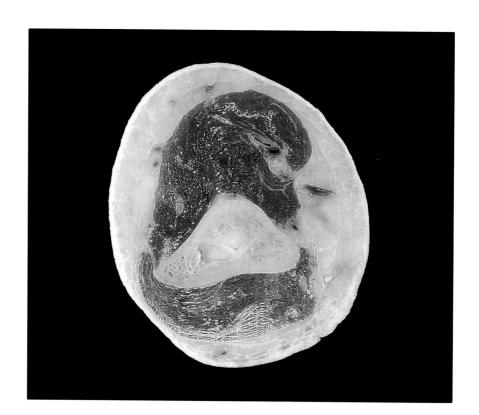

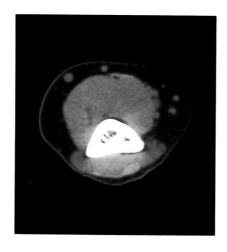

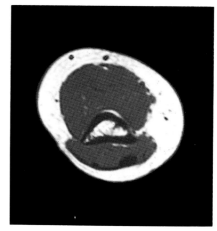

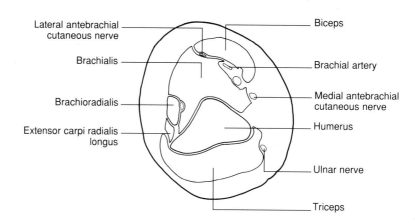

Lateral antebrachial cutaneous nerve

Brachialis

Brachioradialis

Extensor carpi radialis longus

Biceps

Brachial artery

Medial antebrachial cutaneous nerve

Humerus

Ulnar nerve

Triceps

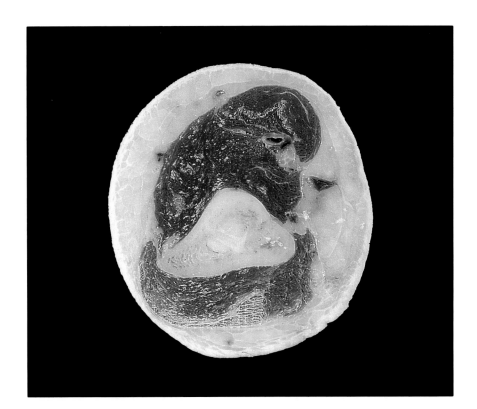

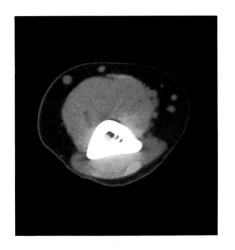
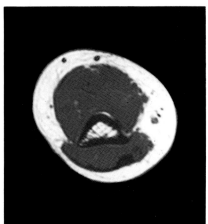

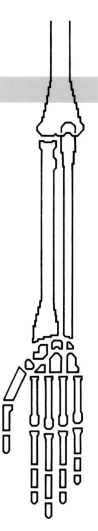

figure 154

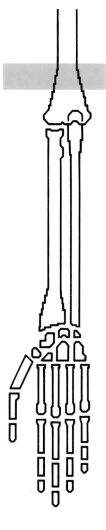

figure 155

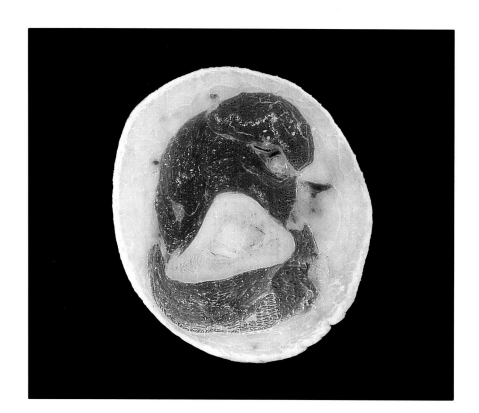

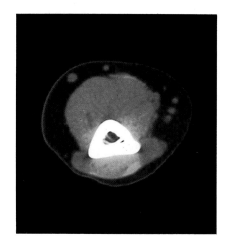

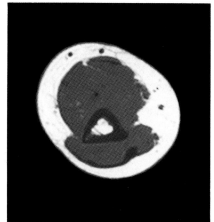

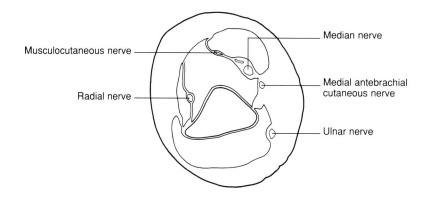

Musculocutaneous nerve

Radial nerve

Median nerve

Medial antebrachial cutaneous nerve

Ulnar nerve

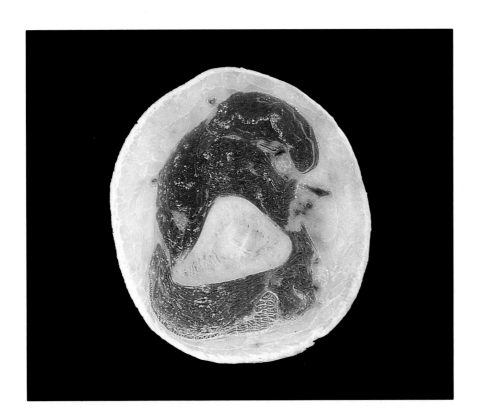

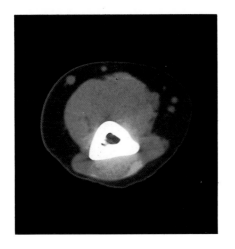

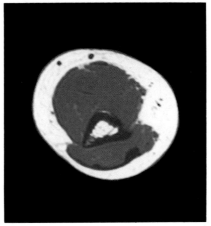

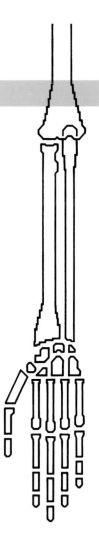

figure 156

figure 157

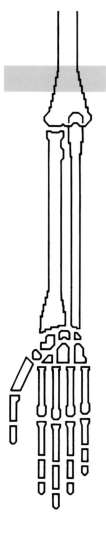

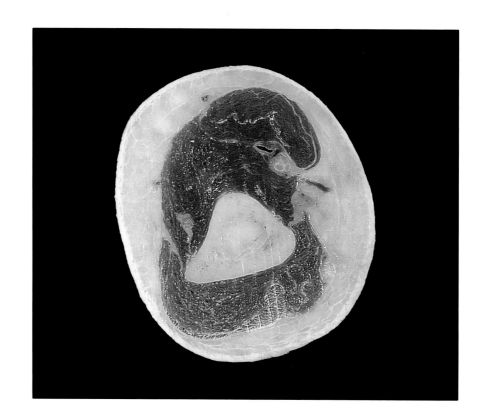

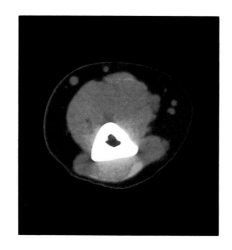

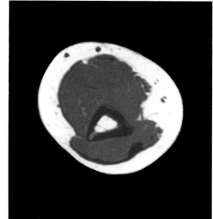

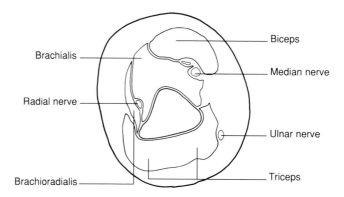

Brachialis — Biceps

Radial nerve — Median nerve

Brachioradialis — Ulnar nerve

— Triceps

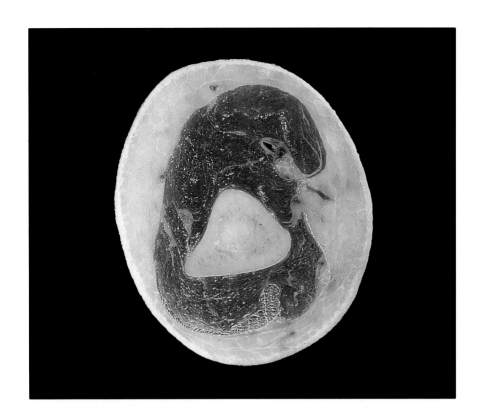

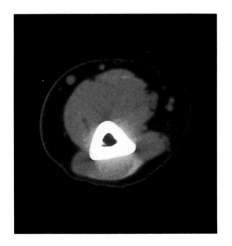

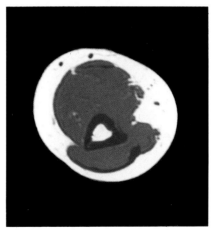

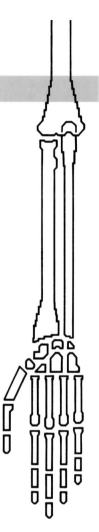

figure 158

figure 159

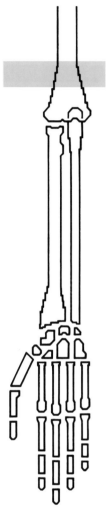

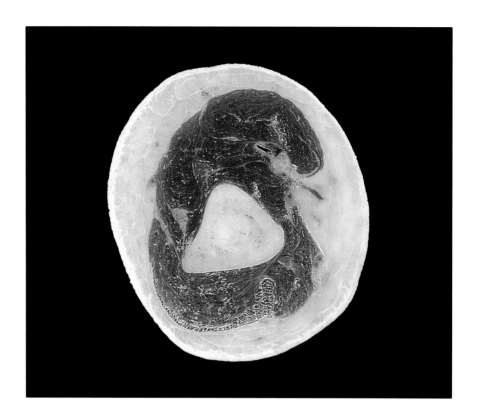

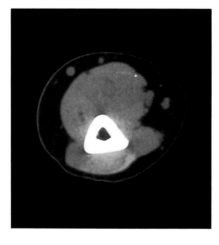

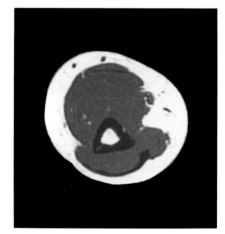

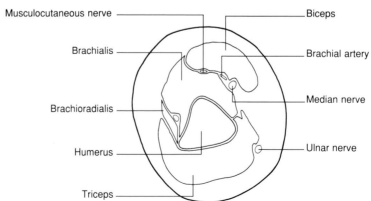

Musculocutaneous nerve — Biceps

Brachialis — Brachial artery

Brachioradialis — Median nerve

Humerus — Ulnar nerve

Triceps

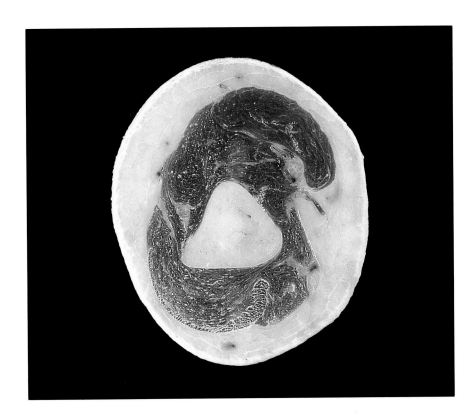

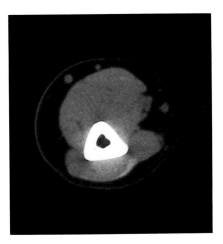

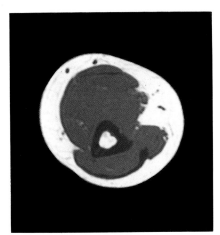

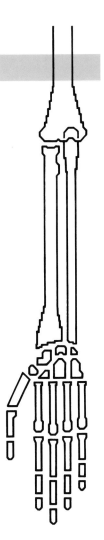

figure 160

figure 161

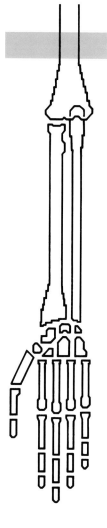

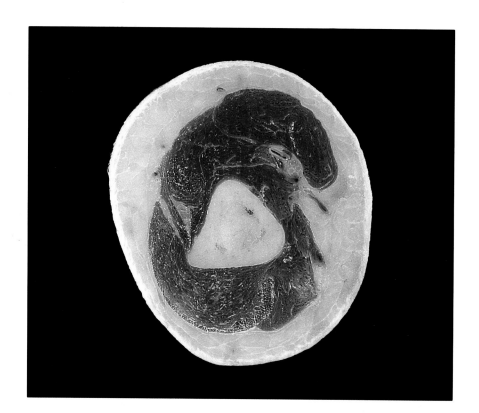

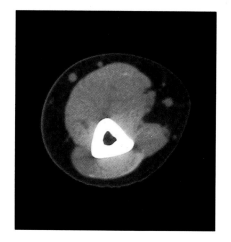

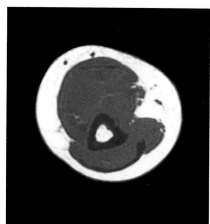

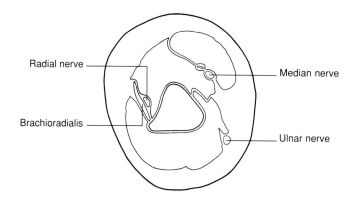

Radial nerve

Median nerve

Brachioradialis

Ulnar nerve

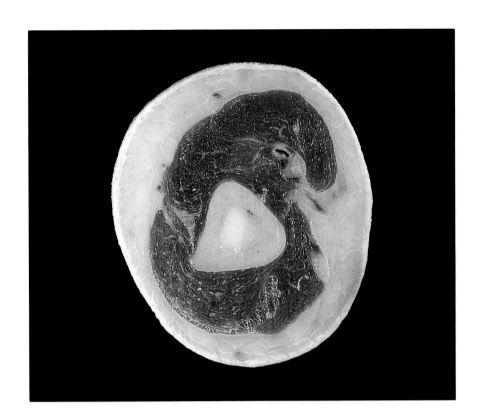

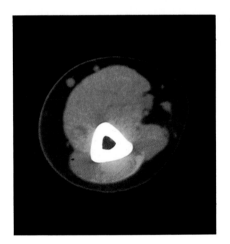
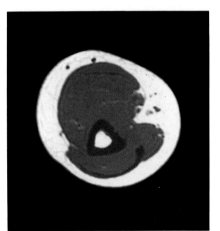

figure 162

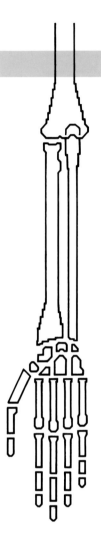

figure 163

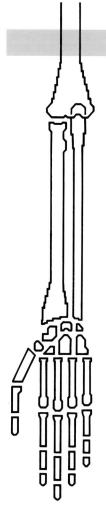

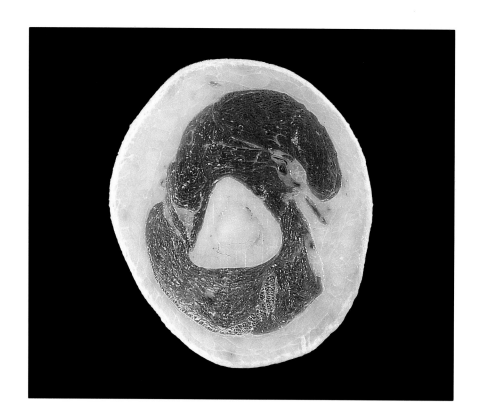

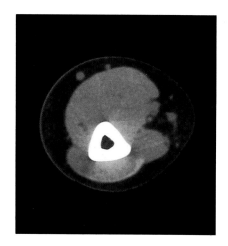

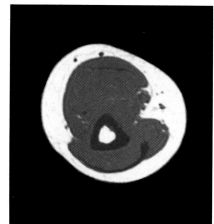

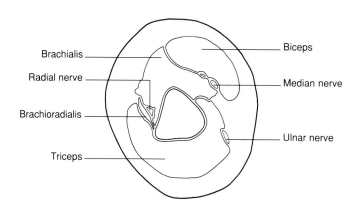

Brachialis		Biceps
Radial nerve		Median nerve
Brachioradialis		Ulnar nerve
Triceps		

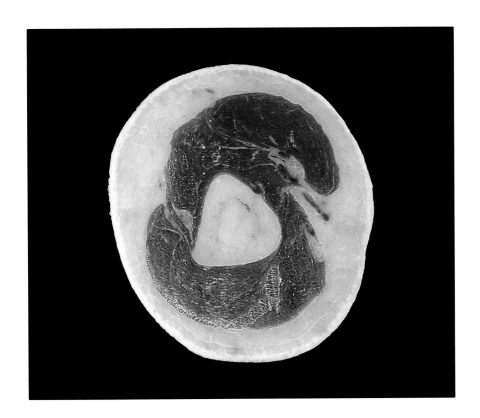

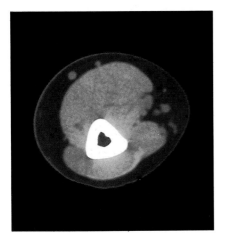

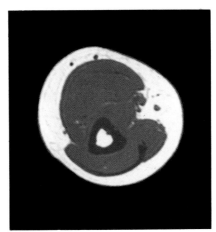

figure 164

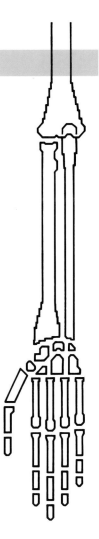

figure 165

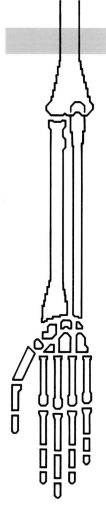

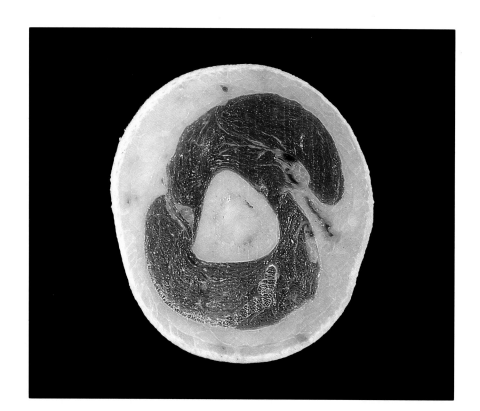

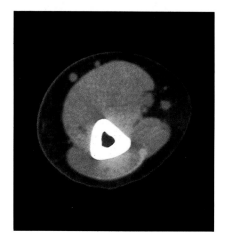

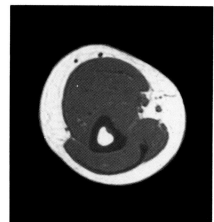

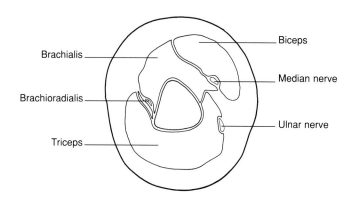

Brachialis

Biceps

Median nerve

Brachioradialis

Ulnar nerve

Triceps

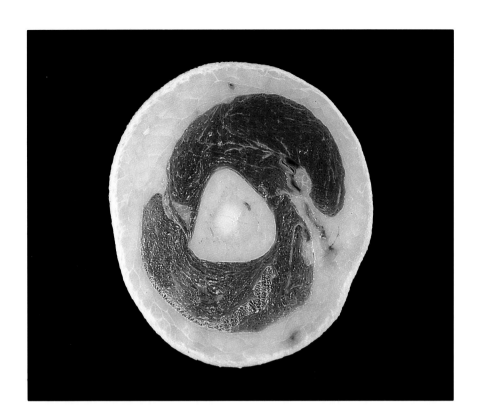

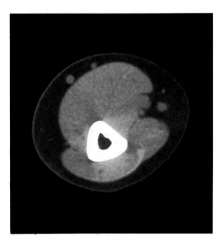

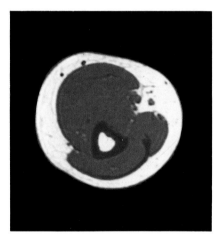

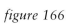

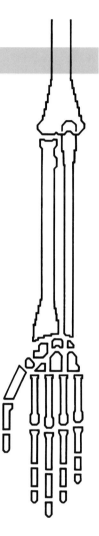

figure 166

figure 167

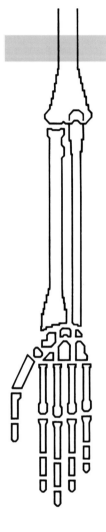

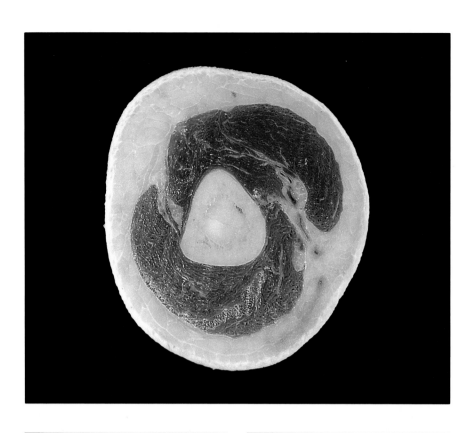

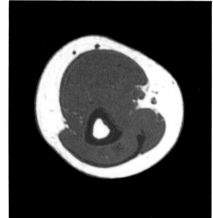

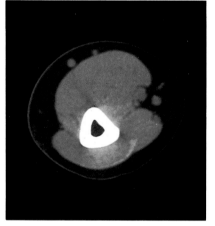

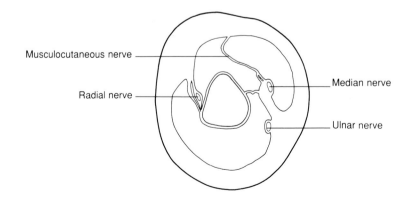

Musculocutaneous nerve

Radial nerve

Median nerve

Ulnar nerve

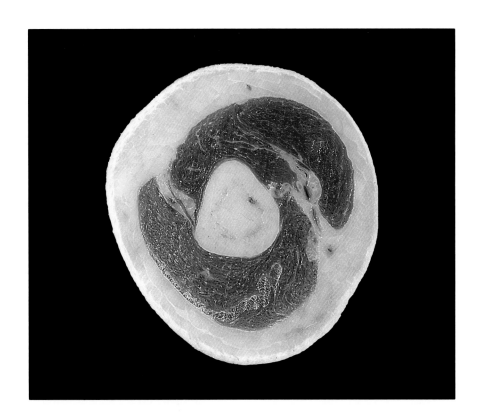

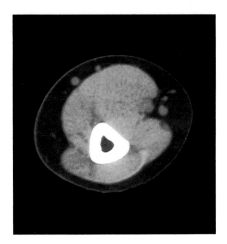 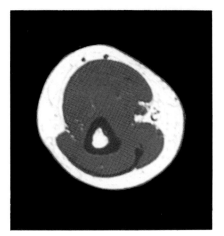

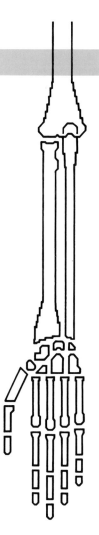

figure 168

figure 169

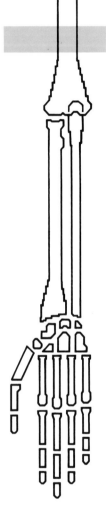

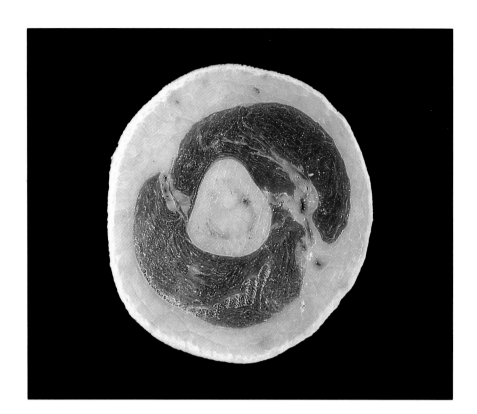

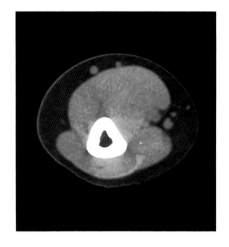

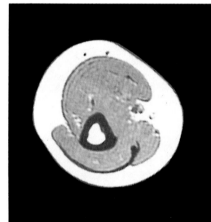

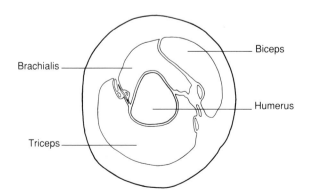

Brachialis

Biceps

Triceps

Humerus

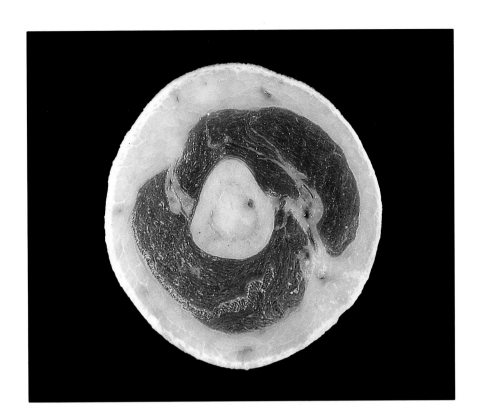

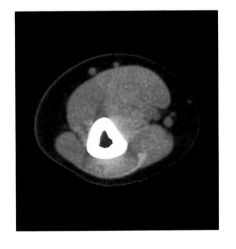 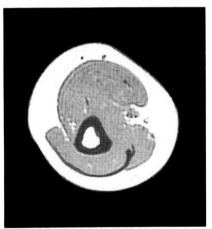

figure 170

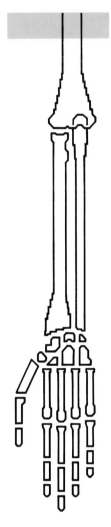

figure 171

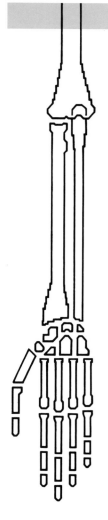

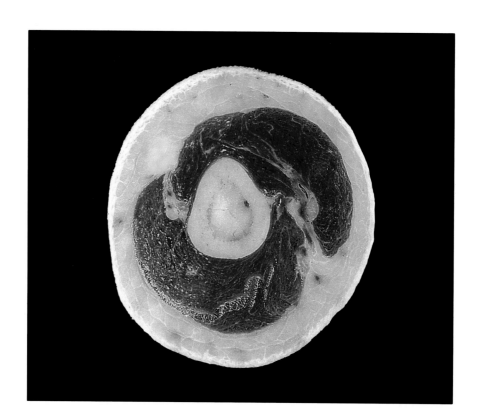

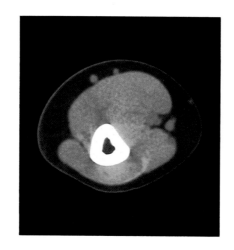

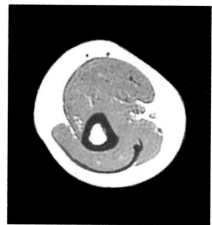

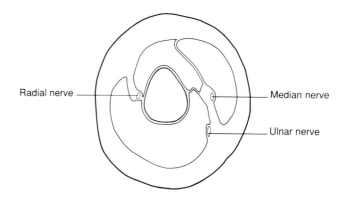

Radial nerve

Median nerve

Ulnar nerve

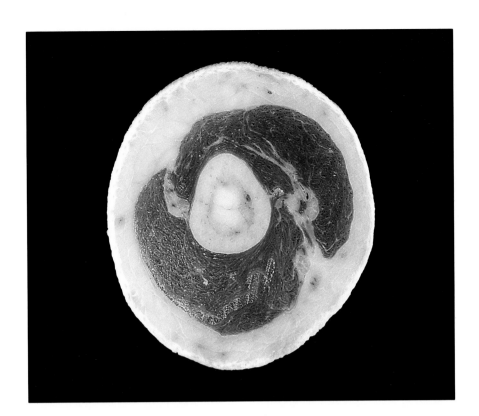

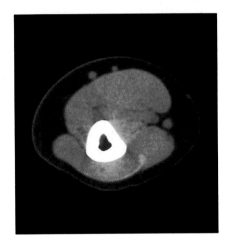

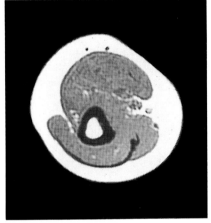

figure 172

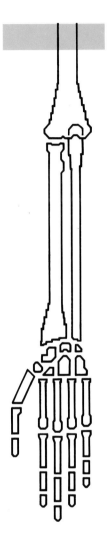

figure 173

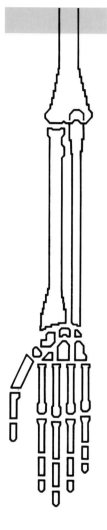

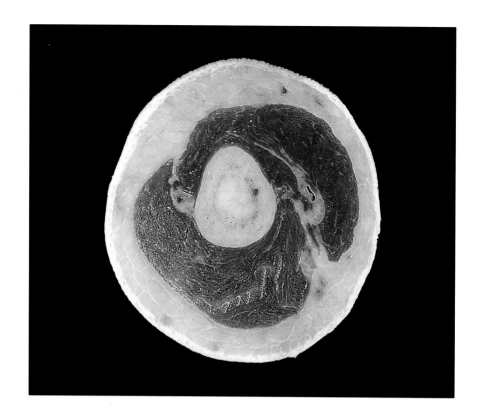

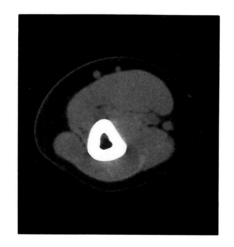

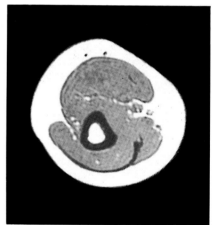

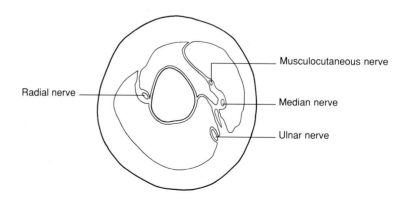

Musculocutaneous nerve

Radial nerve

Median nerve

Ulnar nerve

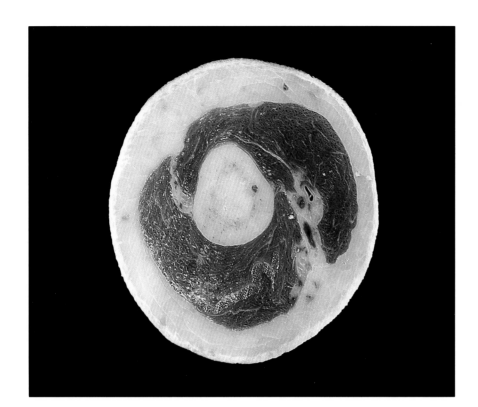

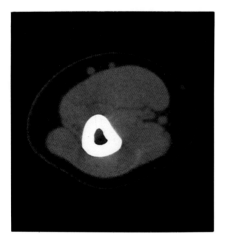

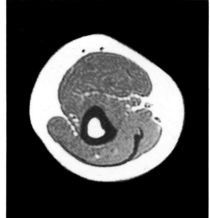

figure 174

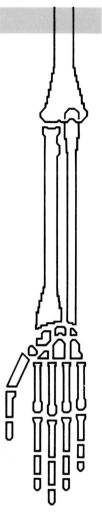

figure 175

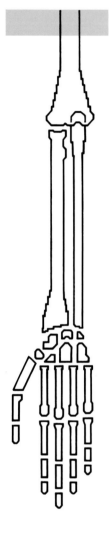

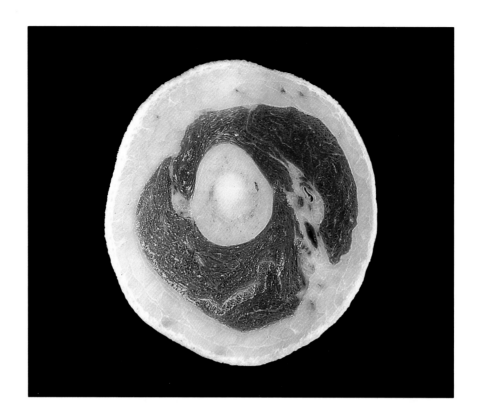

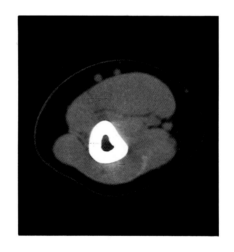

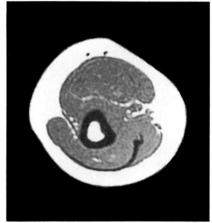

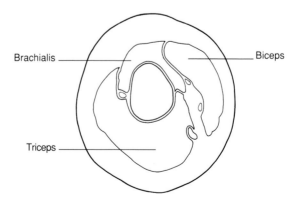

Brachialis

Biceps

Triceps

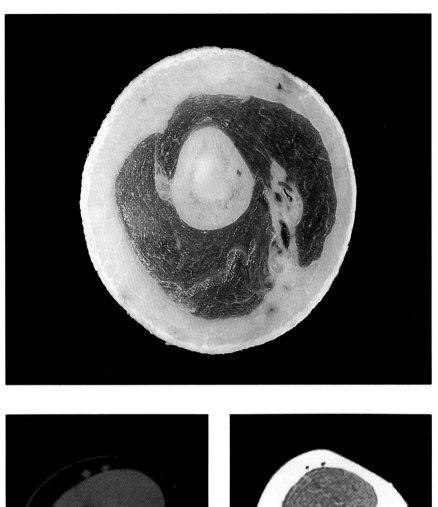

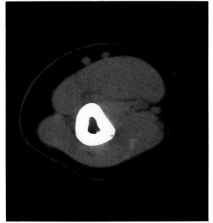
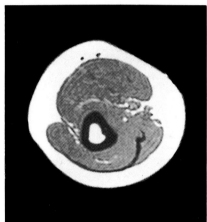

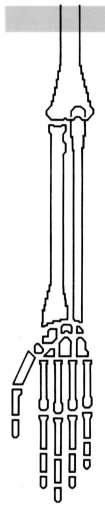

figure 176

figure 177

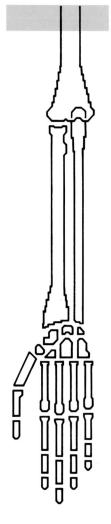

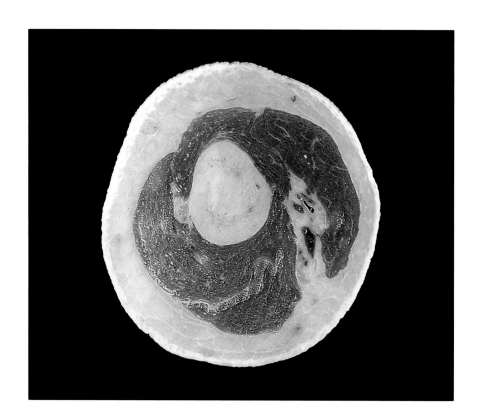

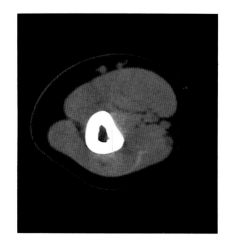

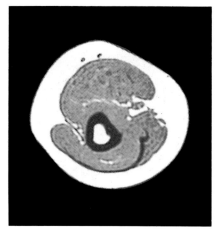

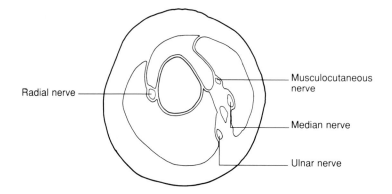

Radial nerve

Musculocutaneous nerve

Median nerve

Ulnar nerve

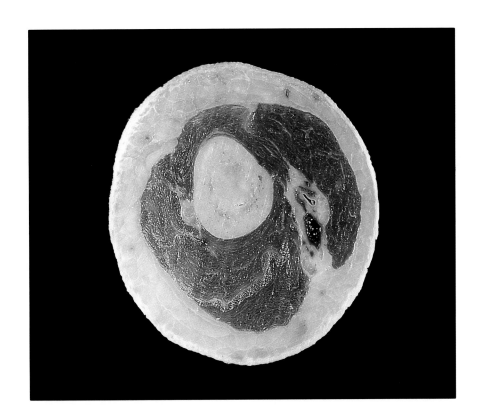

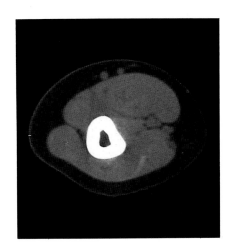

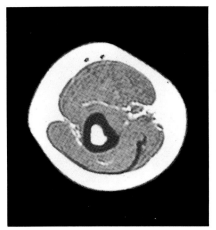

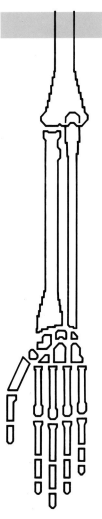

figure 178

figure 179

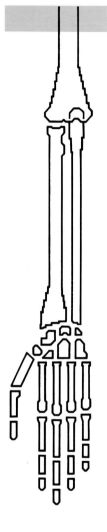

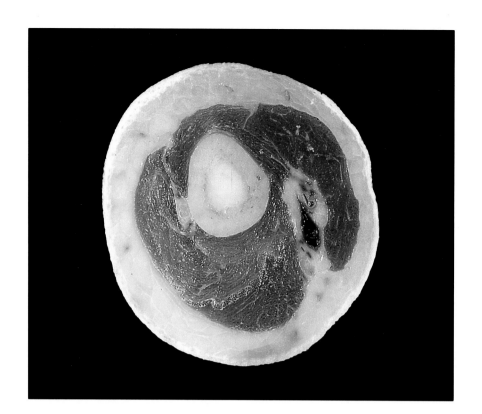

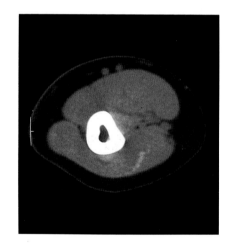

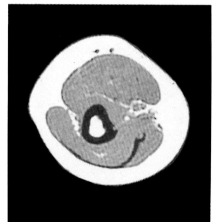

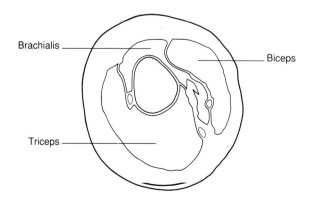

Brachialis

Biceps

Triceps

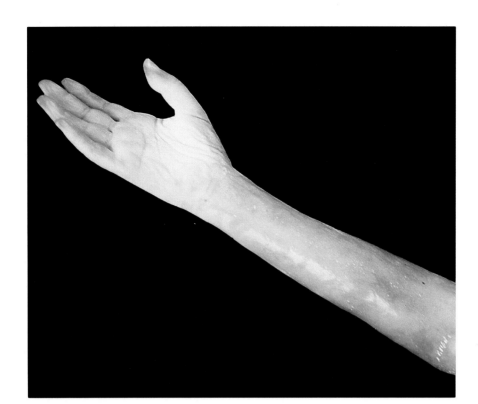

figure 180

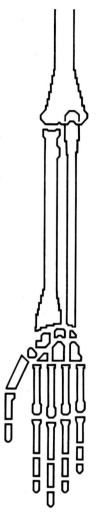